MR. PARKINSON,

LET'S WALK TOGETHER

A Neurologist's Insightful Guide
to Parkinson's Disease and Exercise

JACEY JISEON KIM, M.D.

Mr. Parkinson, Let's Walk Together

Jacey Jiseon Kim

ISBN: 979-8-328-60473-4

First Edition

Printed in the United States of America

RECOMMENDATION

A MUST-READ BOOK ON EXERCISE INFORMATION FOR PARKINSON'S PATIENTS

Beom S. Jeon

- Professor of Neurology, Seoul National University Hospital, MD, PhD
- Specialist in Parkinson's Disease and Movement Disorders, Seoul National University Hospital
- Chairman, World Congress of Neurology (WCN) 2025 Local Organizing Committee
- Editor, Parkinsonism and Related Disorders
- Former President, Asian and Oceanian Association of Neurology
- Former Chairman, World Parkinson's Disease and Movement Disorders - Asia Pacific Section

I have dedicated my life to researching, diagnosing, and treating Parkinson's disease. Meeting patients and caregivers in the clinic, I have noticed some frustrations. One major frustration is that patients often fall prey to unverified information.

Dr. Jacey Kim is a neurologist who specializes in Parkinson's disease. Her extensive experience treating patients and caregivers, combined with her research and deep contemplation, is reflected in this book. It provides accurate knowledge and information about Parkinson's disease with a warm, compassionate touch. Through the stories shared in this book, you will learn about Parkinson's disease and find comfort as well.

I always emphasize exercise in treating Parkinson's disease because it is incredibly important. However, patients often feel lost due to a lack of practical guidance on how to exercise. This book explains the importance of exercise based on research findings and provides realistic exercises that can be easily incorporated into daily life. I believe this book will be extremely helpful, as it is well-written to help patients start exercising with confidence. I highly recommend this book to patients with Parkinson's disease, their caregivers, and the medical professionals who treat them.

RECOMMENDATION

A MESSAGE OF WARMTH AND RATIONAL GUIDANCE FROM A FORMER PROFESSOR

Jong-Min Kim

- Professor of Neurology, Bundang Seoul National University Hospital, MD, PhD
- Specialist in Parkinson's Disease and Movement Disorders, Bundang Seoul National University Hospital
- Director, Korean Parkinson's Disease and Movement Disorders Society
- Associate Editor, Korean Medical Journal

Hearing the doctor say, "You have been diagnosed with Parkinson's disease," can plunge patients into despair. They often wonder if they did something wrong to deserve this or how long they have left to live. The book "Mr. Parkinson, Let's Walk Together," first published in June 2023 in Korean, is a brilliant and practical guide for patients and their families to refer to from the day of diagnosis.

This book is filled with tips that can be applied to daily life. It begins by explaining what Parkinson's disease is and what to expect in the future. It describes in detail what the patient will experience and how treatment will proceed, allowing readers to intuitively understand the disease. As you read further, you will find the core of this book. Look in particular at the chapters "Exercise Slows the Progression of Parkinson's Disease" and "Designing the Right Exercise for Me." They carefully explain the exercises that patients and their families can do, with such kind encouragement and simple direction that they will surely be eager to begin at once. The exercises are not difficult and are presented with warm humor.

This wonderful book is written by Dr. Jacey Kim from Brainup Neurology Clinic. She is a renowned doctor who has cared for many patients at Bundang Seoul National University Hospital and Chungbuk National University Hospital. This book provides warm hope and rational guidance to patients and their families simultaneously. I highly recommend it.

RECOMMENDATION

PARKINSON'S DISEASE AND EXERCISE

Jae-Moon Kim

- Director, Korean Society of Neurology
- Professor of Neurology, Chungnam National University Hospital, MD, PhD

Over 20 years ago, I met a shy and sensitive resident. She had a refreshing charm, like a girl with a rich literary sensibility and a love for beautiful things. After completing her challenging training and enduring the weight of many years, this young doctor has now become an accomplished specialist in Parkinson's disease at a university hospital. Whenever I meet her, I am always impressed by the pure-hearted air of youth that she still retains. While reading this book, I felt Dr. Jacey Kim's warm heart, dedicated to loving and caring for her patients despite her busy schedule.

Many patients in our country believe that most diseases can be treated with good medicine and good food. However, it is crucial to understand that chronic diseases are a part of life that we must learn to live with. Therefore, exercise and discipline that benefit the patient are more important than diet. This book provides daily exercises that can alleviate the symptoms of Parkinson's disease for many patients.

The nervous system is home to many chronic diseases, and since they mostly appear in the elderly, being diagnosed can be alarming. In the clinic, I often tell my patients, "Learn about your disease." Fear grows from ignorance. If you do not know well about the disease you have, it becomes frightening and miserable. Modern medicine cannot cure most chronic diseases completely. Instead, the important task is how to live more happily and healthily while having the disease. Degenerative diseases that appear with aging may feel scarier due to blind anxiety.

This book provides easy-to-understand explanations about Parkinson's disease and details on how patients can live and exercise in daily life. Parkinson's disease affects over 100,000 people in Korea and is increasing globally by more than 10% each year. I believe that after reading this book, you will be well-equipped to overcome the disabilities caused by Parkinson's disease and live a healthier life. Stay healthy and happy.

RECOMMENDATION

EMBRACING LIFE WITH PARKINSON'S DISEASE

Jin-kyu Kim

- Professor Emeritus, Kongju National University, PhD
- Elder, Daejeon Sansung Church
- Former Dean, College of Education, Kongju National University
- Former Dean, Graduate School of Education, Kongju National University

When reading "Mr. Parkinson, Let's Walk Together," I am reminded of a line from the poem "To the Illness" by Ji-hoon Cho:

"Farewell, my friend
Come visit whenever you want
We will talk about life over tea again"

The poem teaches us that no matter how frightening a disease may be, it is about finding peace by befriending the illness rather than fearing it. Parkinson's may still be a terrifying disease in modern medicine. However, Dr. Jacey Kim, the author, strongly asserts that if we have the life force, passion, and love to walk with Parkinson's as a friend, we can overcome it.

The author tells us that treatment is not just what happens in hospitals. Treatment occurs in everyday life, at home, at work, and in all areas of our lives. We must first clearly understand what Parkinson's disease is, including its symptoms, causes, diagnosis, and treatment. Next, we can pursue correct and effective exercise therapies. This book is the fruit of over 20 years of research and treatment by the author, who specializes in Parkinson's disease and movement disorders.

Personally, Dr. Jacey Kim is my daughter. She has always been rational, bold, and deeply caring for others. Recently, the gratitude expressed by those around me who have been treated by her brings me immense joy and pride. It is the grace and blessing of God.

Like smallpox or tuberculosis, Parkinson's disease will someday be easily cured with a simple treatment. I hope that a groundbreaking cure for Parkinson's disease will soon be developed in our medically advanced country. Until then, I hope this book helps you become a friendly companion with Parkinson's disease so that you can happily walk together.

INTRODUCTION

"Ever since I heard I have Parkinson's disease, it feels like my life is falling apart." Parkinson's disease is not an easy condition to deal with. Your hands tremble, and your motor functions gradually decline. However, what might be the hardest part for our patients is probably the stigma of being a "Parkinson's disease patient." The emotional burden that Parkinson's disease carries is immense, oftentimes more than the actual physical discomfort.

I am a neurologist. I specialize in Parkinson's disease and movement disorders, and for over 20 years, I have met many patients and their caregivers. I wanted to convey the correct information about Parkinson's disease that I couldn't fully cover in the clinic.

This book aims to explain what Parkinson's disease is precisely. While it's always said that exercise is crucial for treating Parkinson's disease, there was a lack of detailed guides on how exactly to exercise. Over many years, I have referenced numerous studies and global data, researching and contemplating exercise therapy that patients can do on their own. This book is the result of that effort. Therefore, this book places significant emphasis on how to exercise effectively and correctly for Parkinson's disease.

Treatment for Parkinson's disease isn't just about what happens in the hospital. It's also about what happens in your daily life—at home, at work, and in every aspect of your life. I wrote this book with a lot of thought about how patients can exercise correctly and effectively In their everyday routines.

The book is divided into four chapters.

The first chapter covers the essentials of what Parkinson's disease is, including its symptoms and causes.

The second chapter explains how Parkinson's disease is diagnosed and treated.

The third chapter discusses the importance of exercise in Parkinson's disease, analyzing and summarizing research findings to date.

The fourth chapter is about practical exercise methodologies, explaining specific ways Parkinson's patients can start to engage in effective and beneficial exercise. By looking at patient cases and questions, you can learn about Parkinson's disease and apply exercises that best suit you.

Treatment received in hospitals is crucial, but so is incorporating exercise into daily life. I have written this book to be easy to understand, ensuring that both patients and their caregivers can apply its advice practically. At the same time, the information is backed by solid scientific and medical evidence. My hope is that this book will help not only patients but also the medical professionals treating Parkinson's disease, rehabilitation teams, and caregivers in understanding the condition.

Do you feel like you're alone in a strange place after being diagnosed with Parkinson's disease? This book will be here to accompany you every step of the way.

"Mr. Parkinson, let's walk together."

TABLE OF CONTENTS

PART 1.
OVERVIEW OF PARKINSON'S DISEASE

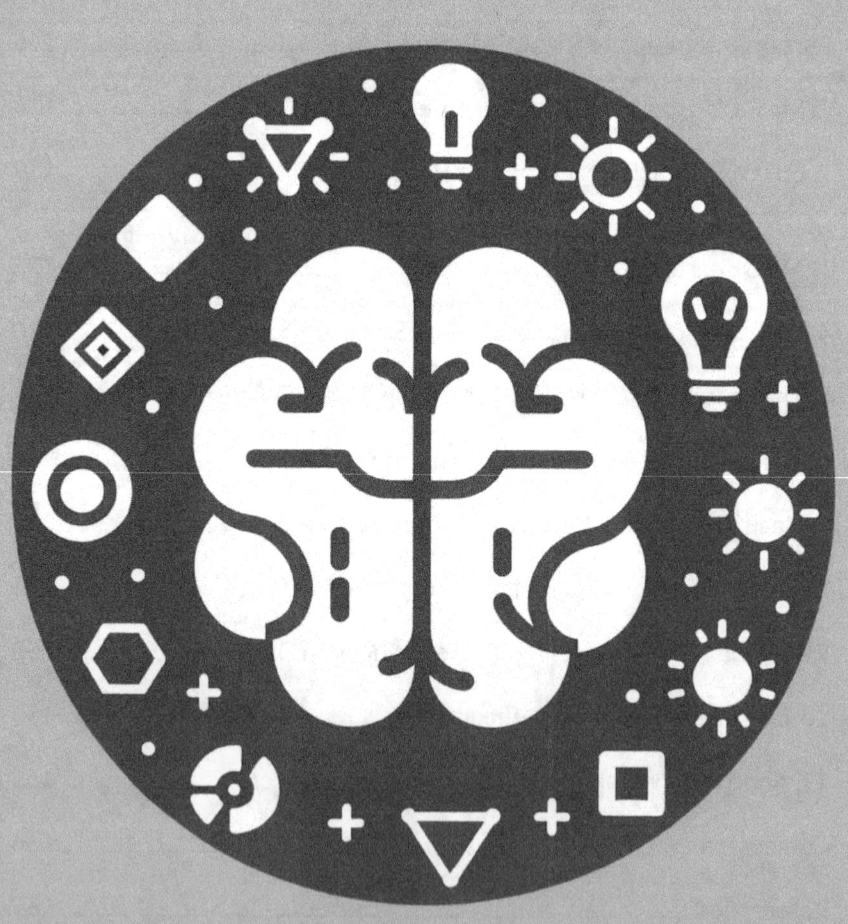

1. JAMES PARK MEETS PARKINSON'S DISEASE

"Mr. James Park , please come in after the current patient leaves."

All my life, I've been called "Doctor," but here at the hospital, I'm always "Mr. James Park ." And whenever I try to ask something, the receptionist is always busy. Holding my appointment slip and waiting for the right moment to ask a question, I think, "This must be how graduate students feel in front of their professors."

The clinic door opens, and an elderly man comes out. Supported by a young man, he has a blank look in his eyes and drool at the corners of his open mouth. Each step he takes seems to be a struggle.

"Mr. James Park, please go in quickly!"

The neurology professor is sitting there. This is my second consultation, and having seen her once, she feels a bit more familiar. To be honest, I was a little surprised when I first saw the neurology professor. I had pictured an elderly man, but she was a young woman, about the age of a mother with a young child.

"Oh, Professor, you look so young."
"Ha ha ha, thank you for saying so. I've already been a neurologist for 15 years."

I regretted blurting that out, but fortunately, she took it well and I felt a bit relieved. How fast time flies, making me realize how much I've aged.

I first noticed "something's wrong with my body" exactly a year ago. I went on a trip to Vietnam with my friends and their spouses. We were all friends who had studied abroad during difficult times and met each other at a research complex after returning to Korea. These friends were my comfort when work at the research institute was tough, and we shared laughs and tears while raising our children together. Before we knew it, one by one, we all retired. When the youngest member of our group retired, we planned a celebratory trip, marking what we called the golden period of our lives. Although I felt my body wasn't what it used to be, I thought, "I've traveled to the US and Europe on tight schedules, so what's a little trip to Southeast Asia?"

On the way to the Korean Air ticket counter after arriving at Incheon Airport, everyone was walking excitedly and quickly, but I couldn't keep up. On one side, I had a golf bag, and on the other, a travel bag. My right leg felt awkward. A junior colleague walking briskly said, "Whoa, did our senior bring a ton of gold in his bag?" and quickly snatched my bag, saying it looked heavy. My right foot couldn't keep up with my left. Throughout the trip, I was constantly worried.

Playing golf for the first time in a long time, I was too tired to keep up with my friends, so I quit halfway. On my way back to the hotel alone, I sat in a cart, leaned back, and looked down at my right hand. My hand was shaking.

The more I searched the internet, the more my symptoms pointed to Parkinson's disease. Thinking "It's just a temporary symptom," I exercised hard and ate good food. In truth, I was afraid of going to the hospital, thinking "What if it's really Parkinson's?" But because of my daughter who came down from Seoul after a long time, I ended up going to the hospital. My daughter was shocked.

"Dad, do you know your hand is shaking?"

She frantically searched her smartphone and called her friends here and there, saying we needed to go to a hospital, and was on the verge of tears, worrying alone.

"I'll take care of it," I said.

And so, I made an appointment at a nearby university hospital's neurology department. Before the appointment, I endlessly searched for symptoms that could be mistaken for Parkinson's disease. I didn't want it to be Parkinson's. I used to chide my wife for being so into church, but now I thought maybe I should have attended church more often and prayed more. Then the result of the first consultation was as expected.

"It looks like Parkinson's disease. We'll do some tests, especially a dopamine PET scan, which will show the level of dopamine activity in your brain. We'll see you again after the tests."

Today is my second consultation; I will check the test results and hear the plan for the future. I hoped until the last moment that the results wouldn't show Parkinson's disease. I hoped the young female professor had made a mistake. But science didn't work that way. There were symptoms, there was reasonable suspicion about the symptoms, and the dopamine PET scan confirmed it. Even when I saw the significantly reduced dopamine activity in one basal ganglion with my own eyes, I hoped it wasn't true.

"Could the image be of somebody else's brain?"
"Should I ask them to check my name again?"

The doctor explained diligently how to take the medication, what side effects to expect, and what to do if those side effects occur. I focused on listening, but all the sounds seemed to fly away into the air. The doctor asked,

"Do you have any other questions?"
"No, I don't. Thank you for your hard work."

I had thousands of questions in my mind, but my mouth said something else. I walked out of the consultation room. It felt like the people waiting for their turn were staring at my walk.

"Ha, so, now I'm a 'Parkinson's patient'?"
"What exactly is Parkinson's disease?"
"Am I going to be completely paralyzed and die?"

"Should I write a will?"
"Life was just starting to get good."
"I won't be able to walk, right?"
"Will I get dementia too?"
"Why? Why did I get Parkinson's disease?"
"How should I live now?"

As soon as I left the consultation room, a cloud of thoughts erupted like a volcano. Soon, tears streamed down uncontrollably. It was the first day I was officially a Parkinson's patient.

2. MR. PARKINSON, WHO ARE YOU?

WHAT IS PARKINSON'S DISEASE?

James Parkinson was born on April 11, 1755, in London, England. The world was quite chaotic at the time with the dawn of the Industrial Revolution and the subsequent struggle for dominance amongst the European powers. James Parkinson, who became a surgeon like his father, was a man knowledgeable in the fields of politics and geology.

"An Essay on the Shaking Palsy"

This is the essay James Parkinson published in 1817. Parkinson, who had excellent observational skills, examined patients with unique symptoms. They had something in common. One arm started shaking, and their movements became very slow. Their shoulders were hunched, and they walked as if they were about to fall forward. They were different from typical paralysis patients. As he closely observed these distinctive patients, he encountered similar people on the streets. They also had shaking arms, appeared to be paralyzed, and had gait disturbances.

Parkinson summarized six cases and published them. At the time, it was an unknown disease without even a name for the condition. As medicine and science advanced, Parkinson's writing received renewed attention. The patients Parkinson examined and observed had the same pathological abnormalities in what turned out to be a degenerative brain disease. Therefore, the disease was named "Parkinson's disease" after the doctor who first described it.

Parkinson's disease is a degenerative brain disease.

Degenerative means gradually fading and dying. Our brains are a mass of neurons, comprising of very tiny nerve cells that are densely interconnected. These nerve cells communicate with each other through neurotransmitters.

One of these neurotransmitters is dopamine. Parkinson's disease is a condition where the nerve cells related to dopamine gradually fade and die. Therefore, in the brain of a Parkinson's patient, dopamine is depleted. Simply put, the dopamine production factories in the brain gradually shut down. What happens to our bodies when dopamine is depleted?

Parkinson's disease is a brain disorder caused by a lack of dopamine.

I think of a puppet show where a puppet is moved by strings attached to its hands. Once, I bought a Pinocchio hand puppet because it looked so pretty at a street stall while traveling. The vendor deftly moved the puppet, making it dance beautifully, but when I tried at home, it looked like a scarecrow's dance. It's because my hands were clumsy and couldn't move the puppet naturally. Dopamine acts like the strings that make the puppet's movements smooth and natural. Dopamine nerve cells form connections that allow us to move elegantly. When dopamine is lacking and the connections don't work well, movements become stiff, slow, and dull. Hands may tremble, and gait may change.

Parkinson's disease is closely linked to dopamine.

When diagnosing Parkinson's disease, a Positron Emission Tomography (PET) scan is used. This test uses a dopamine-specific substance to show how much dopamine activity is present in the brain. In the brain of a Parkinson's patient, dopamine activity is reduced in one or both basal ganglia. Medications used to treat Parkinson's disease are dopamine-based. When taken, they either act as dopamine in our brain or help it function like dopamine.

Did Dr. Parkinson ever imagine that his book would become so important in later years? April 11, James Parkinson's birthday, is "World Parkinson's Day." It's a day to support and comfort Parkinson's patients and their families. And in 2017, 200 years after his book was written, Parkinson's doctors, patients, and scientists worldwide held grand commemorative conferences. Parkinson's passionate observations and records have become a precious piece of history.

3. WHY DID I GET PARKINSON'S DISEASE?

CAUSES OF PARKINSON'S DISEASE

As seen in the previous topic, Parkinson's disease is a neurodegenerative disorder. It occurs as the neurons in the brain gradually degenerate and disappear. In the midbrain, the area called the substantia nigra, dopamine cells decrease. The substantia nigra is black in color. In the brain of a Parkinson's patient, the substantia nigra is discolored, and under a microscope, the neurons here are degenerated and reduced. As the cells that secrete and receive dopamine decrease, our body experiences dopamine deficiency. That is the symptom of Parkinson's disease. Why are the neurons in the substantia nigra dying? Research on the causes is active, but there's no clear answer yet.

Is Parkinson's disease hereditary?

Patients and caregivers are particularly curious about this. In some cases, Parkinson's disease is hereditary. However, most cases are not related to heredity. To determine whether Parkinson's disease is genetic or environmental, "twin studies" are a good research method. There have been epidemiological studies on twins abroad. If a disease has a strong genetic component, twins with similar genes would have a higher likelihood of getting the same disease. In Parkinson's disease, the familial influence was very low.

Therefore, most Parkinson's disease cases are not related to genetics. However, in cases of Juvenile Parkinson's disease where it occurs at a young age, under 40, genetic factors are more relevant. There are also very rare cases of familial Parkinson's disease with specific genetic abnormalities.

Only 5-10% of Parkinson's disease cases are hereditary. If the genetic influence is not significant, what environmental factors could cause Parkinson's disease? Just as heavy smokers have a higher risk of lung cancer, are there risk factors for idiopathic Parkinson's disease? Environmental factors like MPTP (1-methyl-4-phenyl-1,2,3,6-tetrahydropyridine), some pesticides, heavy metals, carbon monoxide, organic solvents, and head trauma can cause Parkinson's disease. However, there is no clear evidence that everyday factors like stress, smoking, drinking, and lack of exercise cause Parkinson's disease.

Research on the causes of Parkinson's disease continues to be published domestically and internationally. Studies on genetic abnormalities and the progression process after onset are still important topics. It may feel like walking through a dark forest, but humanity's steps are gradually approaching the true nature of Parkinson's disease. I believe that in the near future, fundamental treatment and prevention of Parkinson's disease will be possible.

4. MOTOR SYMPTOMS OF PARKINSON'S DISEASE: TREMOR

There are dozens of symptoms associated with Parkinson's disease. These are combinations of characteristic symptoms called Parkinsonism, which include a few distinctive symptoms: resting tremor, rigidity, bradykinesia, postural instability, stooped posture, and gait abnormalities.

James Park's Tremor Story

I've lived my whole life as an atheist, but facing a serious illness, I naturally began to think about religion. Pretending to be reluctant to my wife's urging, I followed her to church. As soon as we entered the church, someone who looked like the pastor's assistant rushed over.

"Oh, Dr. James Park, you came? How's your health? Welcome."

This kind of fuss is exactly why I dislike coming to church.

I smiled faintly and quickly moved away. I sat on a long bench in a corner of the sanctuary. There was clapping and singing joyfully, then we were told to sit and stand a few times before quiet music started playing. Finally, the atmosphere seemed a bit more stable. The service began. And soon, my right hand started trembling. Worried that someone might notice, I quickly grabbed my right hand with my left. My right hand always starts trembling when I'm sitting comfortably like this. So, I try to calm it by squeezing and twisting my wrist. Today, it trembles even more, maybe because I'm nervous. My wife, sitting next to me, sees my trembling hand and holds it. Her tears fall onto my hand. This is embarrassing; everyone can see us. The seat feels very uncomfortable. As soon as the prayer starts, I pull my hand away from my wife. She looks at me with wide eyes.

"My head hurts a bit, I'll step out!"

I quietly stood up and slowly walked out of the sanctuary. My right hand trembles as I walk, and my right leg drags. While everyone inside the church closed their eyes and prayed to their god, I walked out, one arm trembling, one leg dragging. The short distance of fewer than twenty steps felt incredibly long.

'Is God watching this scene?' 'Is this because I didn't believe in you, that you made me like this?'

It felt like being the only kid sent out of the classroom while all the model students stayed in their seats.

Tremor is a characteristic symptom of Parkinson's disease.

The title of James Parkinson's 1817 essay was "An Essay on the Shaking Palsy," which shows how strongly tremor is associated with Parkinson's disease. Parkinson's tremor often occurs when the body is at rest, hence the term "resting tremor." It usually diminishes when the patient moves. Early in the disease, the tremor typically affects only one side of the body but eventually may affect both sides. Tremor can appear in the arms, legs, and jaw, but the hands are most commonly affected. The tremor often looks like the patient is rolling a pill or counting money between the thumb and index finger.

In Parkinson's disease, legs can also tremble. If you experience leg tremor while sitting still, Parkinson's disease should be considered as a potential cause. Tremors can also affect the jaw or tongue.

If you're unsure whether your tremor is a resting tremor, observe if it occurs while walking. We naturally swing our arms when we walk, without consciously thinking about it. If one hand trembles while you're walking, it's likely a resting tremor.

Not all tremors are due to Parkinson's disease. There are many conditions and circumstances that can cause tremors, and Parkinson's disease is just one of them. Conversely, not everyone with Parkinson's disease will experience tremors. There are many patients with Parkinson's who do not have a tremor.

Characteristics of Parkinson's Tremor:

- Occurs when the body is at rest: Resting tremor
- Can affect arms, legs, and jaw
- Leg tremor, especially when sitting, is a strong indicator of Parkinson's disease

---

5. MOTOR SYMPTOMS OF PARKINSON'S DISEASE: SLOWNESS

Dopa Min's Story of Slowness

My name is Dopa Min, and I am 75 years old. I was diagnosed with Parkinson's disease at 58. It took several visits to the hospital to finally find out I had Parkinson's. The first sign something was wrong was a feeling of weakness in my right hand. I struggled to button my clothes, and even dialing numbers on my phone became difficult. Eventually, I found it easier to use my left hand. I also felt a dull pain in my right shoulder and constant neck pain, so I went to an orthopedic surgeon to check for a neck disc issue.

An MRI of my cervical spine showed I had a disc problem, so I had a procedure to treat it. I expected to feel much better afterward, but my hand's movements didn't improve. My handwriting changed, becoming smaller and harder to read. When walking, my right leg seemed to drag. I worried it might be a stroke, so I got a brain MRI, which turned out normal.

Despite this relief, my right hand and leg continued to feel paralyzed. I tried acupuncture and sought out renowned physical therapists to relax my muscles, but the relief was only temporary. I could no longer sew, and even knitting became difficult because my right hand was so slow. Around that time, I experienced a lot of stress, insomnia, and severe dizziness, so I visited a nearby neurologist. That's when I first heard the suspicion of Parkinson's disease.

Slowness is a Core Symptom of Parkinson's Disease

Slowness in movement is one of the hallmark symptoms of Parkinson's disease. Your overall movements become slower, and even fine motor skills become clumsy. In the clinic, doctors may ask you to flip your hand back and forth quickly. Difficulty performing such tasks smoothly and quickly is a telltale sign of Parkinson's.

Slowness is known as bradykinesia. It means it takes longer to start a movement, the movement itself is slower, and the motions are smaller. Facial expressions fade, voices become softer and more monotone, and swallowing becomes difficult, causing drooling. When walking, one arm may swing normally, but the affected arm swings less.

People who once had beautiful handwriting may find their writing becoming smaller and less legible as they continue writing. Difficulty swallowing and slowed walking are also part of this slowness.

Initially, slowness often appears on one side of the body. Many patients think it might be a stroke and undergo brain imaging, or they suspect a disc problem and get spinal images. Early subtle slowness often leads patients to various specialists before a diagnosis is made.

Patients often describe their fingers feeling clumsy on a keyboard, making more typos than before. Typing on a phone, buttoning clothes, or sewing also becomes slower and more difficult.

Slowness affects both small and large movements. When walking quickly, one leg may feel slower, causing a limping appearance. Running can make one side feel unusually heavy.

Research by Dr. Ebert and colleagues shows that Parkinson's patients have slower reaction times and movement times for any given task. The exact pathology of this slowness is unknown, but it might be due to failed signal transmission from the brain's basal ganglia to the cortex.

As dopamine function decreases in the brain, slowness worsens. Dopamine PET scans, which measure dopamine activity, show that the less dopamine absorbed, the more severe the slowness becomes. This scan can help gauge the progression of the disease.

Examples of Slowness in Parkinson's Disease

- Facial expressions diminish, and blinking slows.
- Typing on a phone or computer becomes slower.
- Buttoning clothes becomes difficult with one hand.
- Sewing and knitting become challenging due to slowed hand movements.
- Walking may involve dragging one leg.
- Handwriting becomes smaller and less legible over time.

Movie: "Awakenings"

The 1990 movie "Awakenings" touched many hearts. Dr. Sayer, the protagonist, works at Bainbridge Hospital, which cares for Parkinson's patients. He is a humanist doctor who sees patients as individuals to communicate with, not just as subjects for treatment. He treats patients with great dedication, even those whom others have given up on.

In one scene, a completely immobile patient suddenly catches a ball thrown by Dr. Sayer, only to return to a frozen state immediately after. This gives Dr. Sayer hope that these patients can move. He administers Levodopa, a Parkinson's medication, and the patients start to speak and move. It's a miraculous transformation. Leonard, one of the patients, even finds love and happiness for a time, but the side effects of the medication eventually worsen his condition, and the patients revert to their previous states. Despite the short-lived happiness, the time brought immense joy and precious memories to the patients.

6. MOTOR SYMPTOMS OF PARKINSON'S DISEASE: POSTURAL INSTABILITY AND GAIT DISORDERS

In advanced Parkinson's disease, postural instability and gait disorders are common. Postural instability refers to a loss of balance. Changes in posture accompany this, such as a stooped back and bent joints. Walking patterns change too. Initially, one leg might drag, but as the disease progresses, steps become shorter. Patients may walk with a shuffling gait, their upper body leaning forward, which can lead to falls.

As I try to cross the street, my feet just won't move.

Freezing is when your body suddenly stops moving, like it's frozen in place. This happens as Parkinson's disease progresses, and it feels like your feet are stuck to the ground. For example, when you're waiting at a crosswalk and the light turns green, you might find it hard to take that first step. Freezing often occurs when you're about to start moving, when you change direction while walking, or when you try to go through narrow spaces like an elevator door. This hesitation can occur not just when you start moving, but also as you approach your destination.

In Parkinson's disease, movement becomes more restricted when postural instability and gait disturbances begin. When maintaining balance becomes difficult, it's important to focus not just on medication but also on exercise. From this point on, preventing falls is crucial. Sometimes, severe postural instability and gait disturbances can appear early in the disease. In such cases, it's more likely to be a different type of Parkinsonism rather than idiopathic Parkinson's disease.

Examples of Freezing in Parkinson's Disease

Difficulty taking the first step.
Trouble starting to walk after standing still.
Hesitating and shortening steps when changing direction.
Freezing at narrow doorways.
Difficulty stepping onto an escalator in motion.

7. MOTOR SYMPTOMS OF PARKINSON'S DISEASE: SPEECH IMPAIRMENT AND SWALLOWING DIFFICULTIES

Dopa Min's Story of Speech Impairment

Dopa Min has lived with Parkinson's for 17 years. Dressed in a lovely pink cardigan, she comes into the clinic with her son.

"How have you been? Feeling well?" the doctor asks.

Dopa Min smiles faintly and speaks in a mumbled tone. "People can't understand what I'm saying."

Her son quickly explains, "We celebrated her birthday recently. The whole family came over to celebrate. But my aunts, who hadn't seen her in a while, had trouble understanding her. Her speech has become slurred, and her voice keeps getting softer. They started worrying, thinking it might be a stroke or something. I think it stressed her out."

Dopa Min adds, "I can't sing anymore. My voice won't come out. I used to love singing."

People with Parkinson's disease often experience a reduction in their voice volume and clarity. Some even notice changes in their voice as an early symptom. As the disease progresses, speech can become slurred, and in severe cases, the voice can become so soft that it's hard to understand. Issues with speech and voice are quite common in Parkinson's disease.

The difficulty in speaking clearly is due to the slowed and uncoordinated muscle movements caused by Parkinson's. When we speak, our lips, tongue, facial muscles, and breathing muscles all need to work together smoothly. For a louder voice, the breathing muscles must exert more effort, pushing air forcefully over the vocal cords to create sound. Clear pronunciation requires precise and sustained muscle movements in the face and mouth, quickly transitioning to form the next word. Parkinson's slows down these muscle movements, causing delays. The muscles that need fine control and coordination can easily become fatigued. As the disease progresses, it becomes increasingly difficult for Parkinson's patients to produce sound and articulate words.

Common Speech and Voice Issues in Parkinson's Patients

- Softer voice
- Monotone speech, losing the natural rise and fall of pitch
- Speech may become faster and less clear
- Singing high notes becomes difficult, and the voice may sound hoarse

---

Be Careful with Choking

Similarly, people with Parkinson's often struggle with choking when drinking water or eating food. Many patients tell me that eating a meal is a chore and swallowing pills with water is equally challenging. The muscles in the tongue and face need to work in harmony to chew and swallow food. When swallowing, these muscles must quickly act to prevent food from entering the airway. As these movements slow down and coordination decreases, chewing and swallowing become difficult. Choking can lead to aspiration pneumonia, so it's crucial to be very careful.

When speaking, focus on clearly pronouncing each word. Sometimes, saliva can build up in the mouth, causing a choking hazard. Swallow before speaking. When eating, chew slowly and avoid taking large bites. Talking while eating can overwhelm the muscles in your mouth and tongue. It's better to do one thing at a time.

Start Respiratory Muscle Exercises Early

Respiratory muscle exercises are necessary from the early stages of Parkinson's. Take time to meditate and practice slow, deep breathing . It's okay if your voice isn't strong. Practicing singing loudly is an excellent exercise for controlling your respiratory muscles. When speaking, make an effort to finish your words completely. Parkinson's patients often find their pronunciation and voice fade as they continue speaking. Develop a habit of emphasizing and clearly pronouncing the ends of your sentences.

8. NON-MOTOR SYMPTOMS OF PARKINSON'S DISEASE

James Park's Story: Constipation Is the Hardest Part

"How have you been lately?" my neurologist asked.

"Well, I've been getting by," I replied, giving my usual answer to my al-ways-busy doctor.

"What's been the most challenging for you?"

I hesitated, thinking of giving a vague answer, but then I decided to be honest about what's really been bothering me.
"Honestly, the hardest part lately is going to the bathroom."

At some point, going to the bathroom became a nightmare. I can't even remember the last time I had a comfortable bowel movement. I eat, my stomach gets full, but I don't get the urge to go. My stomach gets more and more uncomfortable, and I feel like I need to go, so I head to the bathroom and try to push. But nothing happens. I strain and strain, sometimes going back two, three, even four times. Some days, I go three times before lunch, three times before dinner, and twice before bed, only to produce tiny amounts each time. The next day, I went to a nearby clinic and was given a laxative. The laxative was so strong that I ended up with diarrhea the following day and spent most of the day running back and forth to the bathroom. After that, nothing for a week. I thought about taking the laxative again, but I worried about becoming dependent on it.

Come to think of it, I had constipation even before I was diagnosed with Parkinson's. I've always taken probiotics, eaten yogurt, prunes, and other foods that are supposed to help with constipation, but it hasn't made much of a difference. After being diagnosed with Parkinson's, I was so focused on my hand tremors that it wasn't until I settled into a routine that I realized how much constipation was affecting me. "Is your constipation severe?"

"Yes. Even when I take medication, it only helps temporarily. Sometimes it doesn't work at all. Is it a side effect of the Parkinson's medication? The Sinemet instructions mention constipation as a side effect."

"Yes, if you didn't have constipation before starting Parkinson's medication and developed it afterward, it could be a side effect. But fundamentally, Parkinson's itself causes many non-motor symptoms like constipation."

Parkinson's Disease and Non-Motor Symptoms

Parkinson's disease is known for affecting movement. It slows down motor functions, makes walking difficult, and causes tremors in the hands and legs. But beyond these motor symptoms, Parkinson's brings a variety of other symptoms, known as non-motor symptoms. In fact, non-motor symptoms are often more varied and severe than motor symptoms. If motor symptoms are the tip of the iceberg, non-motor symptoms are the huge mass of the iceberg hidden beneath the surface.

The Many Faces of Non-Motor Symptoms

The non-motor symptoms of Parkinson's are incredibly diverse. They include sleep disturbances, memory problems, depression, hallucinations, constipation, digestive issues, orthostatic hypotension, and pain. These symptoms don't respond well to traditional Parkinson's treatments like levodopa. Depending on the type and severity of the symptoms, additional tests and different treatments may be needed. For some patients, non-motor symptoms are even more challenging than motor symptoms. What's clear is that non-motor symptoms are an inevitable part of Parkinson's, and understanding them is crucial.

9. IN-DEPTH EXPLORATION OF NON-MOTOR SYMPTOMS IN PARKINSON'S DISEASE

Parkinson's disease comes with a wide range of non-motor symptoms. Let's break them down into a few groups:

- Cognitive and Neuropsychiatric Symptoms
- Sleep Disorders
- Autonomic Nervous System Symptoms
- Other Various Symptoms

Below is a table showing the symptoms in each group:

1. Cognitive and Neuropsychiatric Symptoms

Cognitive decline
Depression, anxiety
Apathy
Impulse control disorders
Hallucinations, psychosis

2. Sleep Disorders

Insomnia
Excessive daytime sleepiness
Severe sleep talking, REM sleep behavior disorder
Periodic limb movement disorder
Restless legs syndrome

3. Autonomic Nervous System Symptoms

Orthostatic hypotension
Constipation
Urinary issues - frequent urination, urgency
Excessive salivation
Sexual dysfunction

4. Other Symptoms

Pain
Sensory abnormalities
Fatigue
Loss of smell
Altered taste

Can there really be this many symptoms? It's already challenging to deal with motor symptoms, and now we have to worry about non-motor symptoms like depression, dementia, and urinary problems? Just reading about all these symptoms might give you a headache. But remember, not all symptoms appear in every patient. Depending on the person, they might experience several overlapping symptoms or hardly any non-motor symptoms at all.

According to Dr. Ji-young Kim's research on non-motor symptoms in Korean Parkinson's patients, the most common issues were nocturia (nighttime urination) and constipation. A staggering 82% of patients experienced nocturia, and 70% had constipation. Memory problems were reported by 66%, restless legs by 62%, anxiety by 60%, and insomnia by 60%. Over half of the patients (58%) felt depressed, 56% had sleep behavior issues, 54% had daytime sleepiness, 54% had urinary urgency, 52% had altered taste and smell, 50% had incomplete bowel movements, and 50% had changes in sexual desire. Less frequent symptoms included delusions, falls, vomiting, incontinence, hallucinations, and double vision.

Cognitive and Neuropsychiatric Symptoms: Does Parkinson's Disease Cause Dementia?

Cognitive decline in Parkinson's includes problems with executive function, memory, language, spatial abilities, and mild forgetfulness. Dementia in Parkinson's differs from Alzheimer's or senile dementia, with more prominent declines in executive function, hallucinations, depression, and mood changes rather than severe memory loss. Cognitive decline significantly impacts the quality of life for Parkinson's patients, increasing caregiver burden and reducing productivity, often leading to nursing home or hospital admissions.

As Parkinson's progresses, medications to improve cognitive function may be added. It's crucial to review and reduce medications that might impair memory. Simplifying the medication regimen can prevent confusion and improve awareness.

Cognitive and Neuropsychiatric Symptoms: Life Feels Too Depressing

Over half of Parkinson's patients experience depression. While it can be mild, severe depression is not uncommon and significantly reduces quality of life, affecting both patients and their families. Depression in Parkinson's can be attributed to two main factors:

The disease itself causes gradual degeneration of brain cells. Neurotransmitters that regulate emotions, including those responsible for mood, become deficient, leading to symptoms like depression, anxiety, and obsessive-compulsive behavior. Observations of patients who felt depressed even before their Parkinson's diagnosis suggest a strong link to brain cell damage.

The psychological burden of being diagnosed with Parkinson's and the physical discomfort and loss it brings. Parkinson's is a progressive disease that cannot be cured with effort alone, and it continues to worsen regardless of one's willpower. This relentless decline can make patients feel helpless and deeply depressed.

Depression Can Be Treated

First, it's important to acknowledge that depression and anxiety are common in Parkinson's disease. These symptoms are not a sign of weakness or a lack of effort. Don't hide your depression or pretend it's not there. Instead, talk to your healthcare provider and seek help. Depression is closely linked to neurotransmitters in the brain, such as serotonin. Therefore, medications that increase serotonin levels can help improve your mood. Treating depression is one of the most satisfying aspects of managing Parkinson's disease.

Depression not only affects your daily functioning but also decreases your quality of life and increases mortality rates. Therefore, appropriate treatment is essential. Remember, you're not alone in feeling this way; depression is a common symptom of Parkinson's disease, and it's important to seek proactive treatment.

Autonomic Nervous System Dysfunction

The autonomic nervous system controls bodily functions that occur without conscious effort. This includes regulating blood pressure, digestion, body temperature, and breathing, whether you're awake, asleep, or even traveling to the moon. In Parkinson's disease, the autonomic nervous system can become dysfunctional. Studies report that 14% to 80% of Parkinson's patients experience this. Autonomic dysfunction can occur at any stage of Parkinson's disease, even before diagnosis. Symptoms vary widely and can include orthostatic hypotension, constipation, urinary problems like urgency and frequency, erectile dysfunction, and excessive sweating.

Cardiovascular Autonomic Dysfunction and Exercise

The most significant factor leading to cardiovascular regulation issues in Parkinson's disease is sympathetic nervous system dysfunction, affecting about 50% of patients. Cardiovascular autonomic dysfunction can manifest as orthostatic hypotension, persistent high blood pressure, and increased heart rate. These symptoms can worsen with Parkinson's medications. Orthostatic hypotension occurs when blood pressure drops suddenly upon standing up, causing dizziness, blackouts, and ringing in the ears. In severe cases, it can lead to fainting and falls, reducing the quality of life. Early diagnosis and management are crucial to prevent falls and other complications from orthostatic hypotension.

Urinary Issues

Urinary problems can arise with Parkinson's disease, including issues like frequent urination, urgent need to urinate, and nighttime urination. Studies suggest that up to 93% of patients experience these symptoms, which can significantly impact social activities. For men, particularly those middle-aged and older, these issues may be compounded by prostate problems, making urination even more challenging. Additionally, urinary problems can severely disrupt sleep, as many patients wake frequently during the night. If sudden urinary issues occur, they may indicate bladder infection, kidney disease, or reproductive organ issues, and it's crucial to get appropriate tests to determine the cause.

If Only I Could Sleep Well

Getting a good night's sleep has always been considered a blessing, and it's something many Parkinson's patients, as well as the general population, struggle with. Insomnia is a common issue, especially as we age, making restful sleep elusive. When was the last time you woke up feeling completely refreshed? In Parkinson's disease, sleep disorders are prevalent, affecting up to 98% of patients. These disorders come in various forms, such as difficulty falling asleep, frequent awakenings, vivid dreams with physical actions (REM sleep behavior disorder), excessive daytime sleepiness, periodic limb movements, and disrupted sleep patterns.

Why Do These Sleep Issues Occur?

The diverse range of sleep problems in Parkinson's disease stems from the overall degenerative changes in the brain. Not only do dopamine-related neurons degenerate, but non-dopamine pathways in the brain also get affected, leading to sleep-related symptoms. Psychological factors like anxiety and compulsions, along with the waning effectiveness of dopamine medications at night, contribute to these issues. When sleep problems arise, consulting a neurologist to identify and manage the underlying causes is essential. Treatment often involves medication to regulate sleep and nonpharmacological approaches like meditation, breathing exercises, and transcranial magnetic stimulation.

One of the hardest aspects of insomnia is the short, poor-quality sleep, and the subsequent "anticipatory anxiety" can further diminish our quality of life. You wake up at 2 a.m. after only a few hours of sleep, use the bathroom, and then lie awake, becoming more alert and anxious about the day ahead. The worry about how difficult the day will be without enough sleep, and the fear of developing dementia from lack of rest, can be overwhelming. Even feelings of resentment towards a peacefully sleeping partner may arise. This anxiety and obsessive need to sleep can be more detrimental than the lack of sleep itself.

It's Okay Not to Sleep Perfectly

I always emphasize to patients that it's okay to think "it's fine" even if you don't sleep perfectly. While it's ideal to sleep soundly like a baby, not everyone can. Our brains are remarkably adaptive and will find ways to get enough rest. Even short naps during the day count as "sleep time" for our brains. Though good sleep is beneficial, not sleeping well doesn't necessarily ruin our lives. Many people naturally have short sleep durations. Efforts should be made to improve sleep patterns, but it's also important not to become overly distressed when those efforts fall short. A more relaxed attitude towards sleep can be beneficial.

Are Your Dreams Vivid?

Parkinson's disease is often diagnosed when motor symptoms, such as tremors or slow movements, become apparent. However, non-motor symptoms can precede these by years. When patients first visit, we ask about non-motor symptoms, as their presence can indicate a higher likelihood of developing Parkinson's later. Three key questions are:

Are your dreams vivid and active?
Do you suffer from constipation?
Have you lost your sense of smell?

Vivid dreams where you physically act out movements, sometimes even falling out of bed, are a condition known as REM sleep behavior disorder. REM sleep is a deep sleep stage during which our muscles should be relaxed. However, in this disorder, muscles can become active, leading to physical actions. This disorder is considered a precursor to degenerative diseases like Parkinson's.

Diagnosis of REM sleep behavior disorder is confirmed through a sleep study, but it can often be inferred through patient interviews. We always ask, "Are your dreams vivid? Do you act out your dreams?" REM sleep behavior disorder can be managed with medication.

Can Constipation Be Managed?

One of the significant challenges for Parkinson's patients is digestive issues, including excessive saliva, difficulty swallowing, gastrointestinal motility problems, constipation, and fecal incontinence. These can occur regardless of the disease's progression, affecting up to 70% of patients.

While constipation is common in healthy adults, its close association with Parkinson's disease has been documented in studies like the Honolulu Heart Study and the Rochester Epidemiology Project, suggesting it can precede the disease by up to 20 years.

Is Constipation Caused by Parkinson's Medication?

This is a frequent question in the clinic. While many Parkinson's medications list constipation as a side effect, it is essential to distinguish whether constipation is caused by the medication or the disease itself. If constipation started after beginning Parkinson's medication, it might be a side effect. However, if it was present before, it is more likely due to Parkinson's disease. It's also crucial not to attribute all digestive issues solely to Parkinson's. For instance, one of our patients suffering from chronic constipation was later diagnosed with colon cancer during a routine colonoscopy. Regular health check-ups are essential, especially for middle-aged and older adults.

10. NON-MOTOR SYMPTOMS OF PARKINSON'S DISEASE: A CASE STUDY

Help Me Chase Away the Ghosts: The Story of Dopa Min

Dopa Min and her son came to the clinic before their scheduled appointment.

"You're here earlier than expected. Is something wrong?" I asked.

Dopa Min looked noticeably thinner.

"Recently, my mother hasn't been able to sleep at all," her son explained. Ms. Min was experiencing hallucinations. One time, she entered the bathroom on tiptoes, saying the floor was covered with ants. She sometimes saw her deceased cousin. Recently, things had gotten worse.

"Every night, she sees a scary goblin waving a club in the room," her son continued.

Dopa Min would scream at the goblin to leave and swing a pillow at it. She even fell out of bed trying to avoid the goblin's club.

"One night, I heard a commotion and found her hiding behind the curtain, terrified of the goblin," her son said.

The goblin visited every night, causing her to consider asking her church pastor for prayers or using a talisman. Her lack of sleep and overwhelming fear left her too weak to eat.

> "Am I going crazy, or am I possessed by a ghost?"
> "Ms. Dopa Min, your symptoms are called 'hallucinations.'"
>
> Hallucinations mean seeing things that aren't there. People with Parkinson's disease can experience hallucinations.
>
> "It's not because you're mentally ill or possessed by a ghost. It's just a symptom that occurs because nerve cells in your brain are dying."

Hallucinations can take various forms, from seeing small insects to deceased loved ones. Sometimes, unknown individuals appear, talking and acting as if they were real. Patients need to understand these are mere hallucinations, not reality. If you experience such symptoms, think, "This is my Parkinson's causing hallucinations," and discuss it with your doctor.

While not all hallucinations require aggressive treatment, if they severely disrupt daily life and cause extreme fear, as in Dopa Min's case, active treatment is necessary. Emotional support from family and faith is helpful, but it cannot replace the need for addressing the brain's neurotransmitter pathway damage.

Antipsychotic medications are used to manage hallucinations. However, some antipsychotics can worsen Parkinson's motor symptoms, making it a delicate balance. Increasing dopamine-related medications can heighten psychotic symptoms, while increasing antipsychotics can worsen Parkinson's symptoms.

What should be done? Prioritize based on the patient's symptoms. In Dopa Min's case, using antipsychotic medication to reduce anxiety and sleep disturbances, thereby improving her quality of life, was essential. Fortunately, there are antipsychotics that have minimal impact on Parkinson's symptoms.

> Dopa Min's treatment involved adjusting her Parkinson's medication slightly and adding an antipsychotic. Three days later, she returned much calmer.

"The goblin still comes, but its red face is faint, and it's much gentler. Dr. Kim, you really are good at chasing away ghosts," she said.
"Yes, indeed. Parkinson's doctors can be quite effective at chasing away ghosts," I replied.

PART 2.
DIAGNOSIS AND TREATMENT OF PARKINSON'S DISEASE

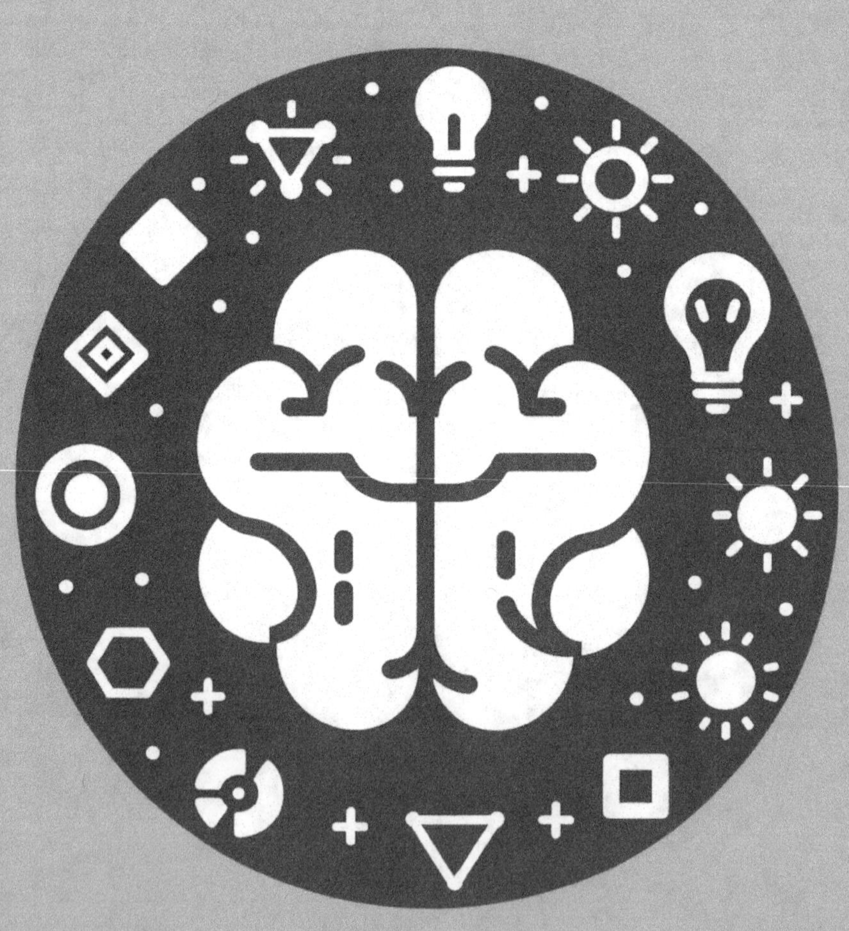

1. DIAGNOSIS OF PARKINSON'S DISEASE

How is Parkinson's Disease Diagnosed? The Story of James Park

When I first heard that my symptoms resembled Parkinson's disease, I couldn't sleep at night. The more I searched online, the clearer it became that my symptoms matched. Should I go to a major hospital? Should I find the most renowned specialist in Seoul? Would the diagnostic methods be the same everywhere? I worried they might run a bunch of unrelated tests.

"How is Parkinson's disease diagnosed?" I wondered.

I made an appointment at the neurology department of a nearby university hospital. On my first visit, I was eager to learn about my symptoms and how Parkinson's disease is diagnosed.

"When Parkinson's disease is suspected, how is it confirmed?"
"Is a brain MRI necessary? Why is it done?"
"If my brain MRI is normal, does that mean I don't have Parkinson's?"
I worried I was asking too many questions but decided to ask everything I was curious about.

The diagnostic process and tests for Parkinson's disease are nearly identical for neurologists specializing in Parkinson's. In this chapter, I'll share the diagnosis process and its significance.

First, let's clarify some terms:

Parkinsonism, idiopathic Parkinson's disease(IPD), Parkinsonian syndrome, Parkinson plus... there are many terms.

Parkinsonism refers to any condition that presents Parkinson's symptoms, such as slowness, tremors, stiffness, and balance issues. Regardless of the cause, these symptoms are collectively called Parkinsonism.

IPD is the most common form, caused by the gradual degeneration of the brain.

Parkinsonian syndrome or Parkinson plus refers to conditions similar to Parkinson's disease but with different causes and prognoses.

The diagnosis of Parkinson's disease involves three steps:

1. Are there Parkinson's symptoms?
2. Is there a cause for the Parkinson's symptoms? (This step involves identifying diseases that cause Parkinson-like symptoms but are not Parkinson's disease.)
3. Is it IPD or another type of Parkinsonism?

Step One: Identifying Parkinson's Symptoms

When a patient comes in with symptoms, the most crucial aspect is the neurologist's examination to determine if Parkinson's symptoms are present. This is the first and most vital step in diagnosing Parkinson's disease.

In medical school, my neurology professor said, "You can diagnose Parkinson's disease from the moment the patient walks into the office."

From the moment a patient opens the door and sits down, I observe every movement. I check for facial expressions, posture, dragging feet, and trembling hands. I also look at their facial expressions and blinking during the consultation. Listening to the patient's history and asking many questions is also a vital part of the process.

After years of treating Parkinson's, I can often tell if a patient has Parkinson's disease just by watching them walk into the room, sit down, and look at me. Sometimes, I even recognize it in people I see on the street.

James Parkinson, who first described the disease, did the same. He meticulously observed patients' movements and even included observations of people he encountered on the streets. Despite over 200 years of medical advancements, the most critical aspect of diagnosing Parkinson's disease remains the neurologist's direct examination of the patient. Observing from head to toe, performing neurological examinations, and checking for various motor signs to confirm the presence of Parkinson's symptoms is the starting point of the diagnosis.

Step Two: Determining the Cause of Parkinson's Symptoms

Even if Parkinson's symptoms are present, it doesn't always mean it's Parkinson's disease. Many conditions can cause Parkinson's symptoms. The most common is IPD, caused by the gradual death of dopamine cells in the brain. However, other causes can lead to secondary Parkinsonism. Identifying these secondary causes is crucial because their outcomes can differ significantly from IPD.

What are the Secondary Causes of Parkinsonism?

Some medications can deplete dopamine levels, leading to Parkinson's symptoms. When these symptoms arise after taking such medications, it's called "drug-induced parkinsonism." This is why it's crucial to check what medications a patient has taken previously. If Parkinson's symptoms are due to medication, stopping the drug can often resolve the issue. So, if you're visiting the hospital for a Parkinson's diagnosis, make sure to bring a detailed list of all the medications you're taking.

Strokes or reduced blood flow in the brain can also cause walking difficulties and slow movements, symptoms associated with "vascular parkinsonism."

The brain contains structures called "ventricles" that are filled with cerebrospinal fluid. When these ventricles enlarge, it's referred to as "hydrocephalus," which can also present Parkinson's-like symptoms.

Other causes of Parkinson's symptoms include having had encephalitis, exposure to toxins, trauma, and carbon monoxide poisoning.

To determine the cause of Parkinson's symptoms, a variety of tests may be conducted. These can include blood tests, autonomic nervous system tests, cognitive function tests, brain MRI, dopamine PET scans, and, if necessary, genetic tests or electroencephalography.

Secondary Causes of Parkinsonism:

Drug-induced Parkinsonism
Vascular Parkinsonism
Hydrocephalus
Infections, toxins, trauma, carbon monoxide poisoning, etc.

Step Three: Determining the Type of Parkinson's Disease

The second step in diagnosing Parkinsonism involves identifying secondary causes. Often, Parkinsonism appears without any specific cause, which is then attributed to degenerative changes in the brain, known as primary Parkinsonism. The third step is determining which type of primary Parkinsonism it is.

The most common type is IPD. There are also 'Atypical Parkinsonism' or 'Parkinson Plus Syndromes,' which have similar but slightly different symptoms and anatomical changes. These include Multiple System Atrophy, Progressive Supranuclear Palsy, Dementia with Lewy Bodies, and Corticobasal Syndrome. These conditions share Parkinson-like symptoms but also have unique features, often referred to as Parkinson Plus. You can find detailed characteristics of each disease in Chapter 3.

Primary Parkinsonism Causes

- Idiopathic Parkinson's Disease (IPD)
- Multiple System Atrophy (MSA)
- Progressive Supranuclear Palsy (PSP)
- Dementia with Lewy Bodies (DLB)
- Corticobasal Syndrome (CBS)

2. THE DIAGNOSIS PROCESS AND VARIOUS TESTS

First Visit to the Clinic

During the first visit, we discuss the patient's medical history and conduct a neurological examination, including the Unified Parkinson's Disease Rating Scale (UPDRS), and review their medication history. If Parkinsonism is suspected, the following tests are performed:

Tests for Diagnosing Parkinson's Disease

- Brain MRI
- Dopamine PET Scan
- Autonomic Nervous System Tests
- Blood Tests, Genetic Testing (for some)
- Cognitive Function Tests
- EEG, Electromyography/Nerve Conduction Studies

Based on the neurologist's examination and test results, we confirm if the symptoms are due to Parkinsonism. If confirmed, we identify the type of Parkinson's disease and its severity. Several tests help in making a more precise diagnosis. Here are explanations of these tests:

- Brain MRI: IPD usually shows a normal MRI, especially in the early stages. MRI is essential to rule out secondary causes like ischemic changes, brain injury, or unnoticed past strokes.

- Dopamine PET Scan: This measures dopamine activity in the brain. IPD shows reduced dopamine activity due to selective death of dopamine cells. Symptoms on the right side of the body correlate with lower activity in the left basal ganglia on the scan. Dopamine PET can detect abnormalities even in early stages, as symptoms appear when over 70% of dopamine cells are lost. This scan helps distinguish between different causes of Parkinsonism; for example, drug-induced or vascular Parkinsonism shows a normal dopamine PET scan.

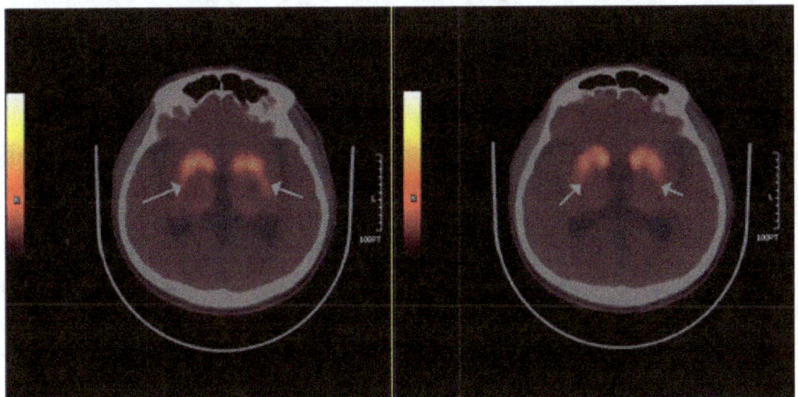

The dopamine PET scan of a Parkinson's disease patient shows reduced dopamine activity in the basal ganglia (indicated by the arrow).

- Blood Tests: Issues with thyroid or copper metabolism can cause tremors or slowed movements.

- Autonomic Nervous System Tests: Parkinson's Disease and Parkinson Plus Syndromes often impair autonomic functions. In Parkinson Plus Syndromes, autonomic dysfunction can appear early, helping in differentiation and assessing severity. Tests include blood pressure measurements upon standing, Valsalva maneuver, heart rate response to standing, and deep breathing.

- Neurocognitive Tests: Parkinson's patients have a higher risk of cognitive decline and dementia. Early mild cognitive impairment can progress to dementia. Neurocognitive tests assess current cognitive function and provide a baseline for future comparison. Depression and anxiety levels are also checked.

- Electromyography/Nerve Conduction Test: These tests measure tremor severity and detect peripheral nerve abnormalities if sensory issues are present.
- Other Tests: EEG and heart scans may be conducted to differentiate from other conditions.

Genetic Testing

Several abnormal genes associated with Parkinsonism are known. It's not feasible to test for all genetic abnormalities in everyone, so we selectively test individuals with a higher likelihood of genetic issues. Most Parkinson's Disease diagnoses occur after age 50, making genetic causes less likely, so genetic testing is often skipped. About 30% of cases occur in those under 50; juvenile Parkinsonism appears before 20, and early-onset Parkinsonism appears between 20 and 40. Younger onset typically indicates a stronger genetic predisposition, warranting family history review and specific genetic testing.

3. TYPES OF PARKINSON'S DISEASE

"Dr Kim, let me tell you something. About five years ago, my hands started shaking, so I went to the hospital. They diagnosed me with something... what was it? Oh, right, Pakistan.., Pakistan disease? What is it?"

"And then my friend asked me, 'There are different types of Parkinson's, right? So, which type do you have?'"

"Suddenly, I became a Pakistan's expert. The term 'Parkinson' is quite challenging. Parkinson's itself is tough, and there are many other terms related to it, making it even more confusing."
"There are many types of Parkinson's disease. Parkinsonism, Parkinson's syndrome, Parkinson's disease, atypical Parkinsonism... Even for doctors who aren't neurologists, categorizing these is not easy because the names and concepts are complex. Each type has slightly different symptoms, progression, and sometimes different treatments."

There are many types of Parkinson's disease. The diagnostic process explained in the previous chapter helps determine the type of Parkinson's one has. You don't need to know every condition that presents with Parkinsonism. However, understanding the basics and knowing your specific type helps you better understand your symptoms. This chapter explains how Parkinson's is categorized and the characteristics of each type.

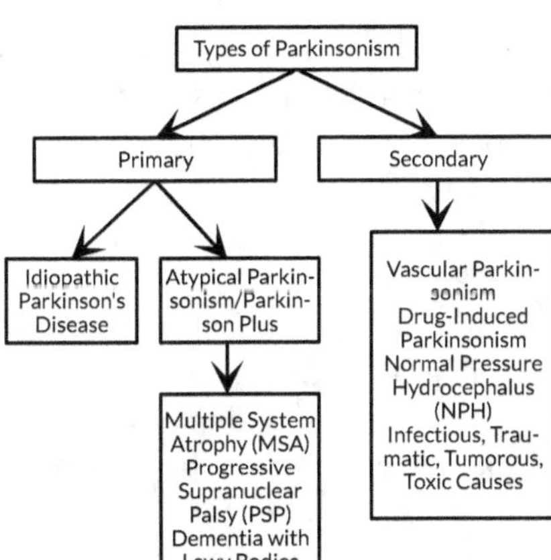

First, Parkinsonism refers to the symptoms of Parkinson's disease and also to all diseases that exhibit these symptoms.
Parkinsonism includes symptoms such as tremors, slowness, rigidity, and postural instability. If these symptoms are present, we call it Parkinsonism.

Parkinsonism can appear in various medical conditions. It can be temporary or indicative of a disease. So, what diseases exhibit Parkinsonism? There are so many that we categorize them into primary Parkinsonism and secondary Parkinsonism.

Second, Primary Parkinsonism, or Parkinson's disease, occurs gradually and progressively as degenerative changes occur in the brain. The most representative type of primary Parkinson's disease is "Idiopathic Parkinson's disease(IPD)." This is the most common and typical form of Parkinson's. When we say "Parkinson's disease," we usually mean IPD.

However, there are other forms of Parkinsonism caused by brain degeneration that are slightly different from IPD. These include diseases like multiple system atrophy, progressive supranuclear palsy, Lewy body dementia, corticobasal syndrome , and spinocerebellar ataxia.

These conditions are similar to IPD but have different symptoms, so they are called Parkinson-plus syndromes, atypical Parkinsonism, or Parkinsonism syndromes. While the definitions vary slightly, these are all forms of primary Parkinsonism excluding IPD.

Third, secondary causes can also lead to Parkinsonism.

While primary Parkinsonism results from gradual and continuous brain degeneration, secondary Parkinsonism has other underlying causes. Parkinsonism can develop after a stroke or brain hemorrhage and can also be caused by conditions such as hydrocephalus, encephalitis, brain injury, traumatic brain injury, tumors, or exposure to toxic substances. If the cause of secondary Parkinsonism is addressed, the Parkinsonism symptoms may improve.

Here are some common diseases that show Parkinsonism:

- Idiopathic Parkinson's disease(IPD): This is the typical form of Parkinson's disease that we commonly refer to.
- Vascular Parkinsonism: Caused by cerebrovascular diseases such as strokes or brain hemorrhages, leading to Parkinsonism.
- Drug-induced Parkinsonism: This type of Parkinsonism occurs after taking certain medications, particularly those that inhibit dopamine.
- Multiple System Atrophy: Early symptoms include autonomic nervous system abnormalities, dizziness, ataxia, and unsteady walking.
- Progressive Supranuclear Palsy: Early symptoms include gait disturbances. While IPD usually causes a forward-leaning posture, progressive supranuclear palsy may cause a backward-leaning posture. Neurological exams may show restricted eye movement.
- Lewy Body Dementia: If dementia develops within a year, Lewy body dementia is a strong possibility.
- Corticobasal Degeneration: Symptoms include tremors, rigidity, and bradykinesia with significant asymmetry. Muscle jerks, dystonia, and apraxia may also be present.
- Spinocerebellar Ataxia: Characterized by cerebellar atrophy on brain MRI and early balance and gait disturbances.

Can the diagnosis of Parkinson's disease change?

"I was diagnosed with Parkinson's disease three years ago. But recently, my diagnosis was changed to Atypical Parkinsonism or Parkinson Plus. Was the original diagnosis wrong?"

IPD and Atypical Parkinsonism can be very similar, especially in the early stages, making them difficult to differentiate. As the disease progresses, the distinctive features of each condition become clearer. Additionally, Atypical Parkinsonism shares some overlapping characteristics and pathological changes in the brain. Since it's impossible to predict the future course of the disease or diagnose by dissecting the brain initially, it can be challenging to accurately diagnose the type of Parkinson's disease early on. Therefore, continuous medical follow-up is necessary to observe medication response, disease progression, and symptom patterns, which help clarify the diagnosis. In some cases, the diagnosis may change. Although the prognosis varies by disease type, treatment is generally similar. Therefore, even if the exact type of Parkinson's disease is unclear, there's no need to worry. Effective treatment is available.

4. PARKINSON'S DISEASE TREATMENT: MEDICATION

"Can Parkinson's disease be treated?"

Upon being diagnosed with Parkinson's disease, the primary concern is treatment. People often wonder whether it is treatable, what medications are needed, and whether they must take them for life. Although Parkinson's disease cannot be completely cured, there has been significant progress in the treatment of Parkinson's disease over the past 50 years, with innovative drugs and surgical methods developed. Don't be discouraged by the inability to cure Parkinson's disease. With medication, symptoms can be managed effectively, and patients can live well. Modern medicine has significantly improved the quality of life for Parkinson's patients.

Medications for Parkinson's Disease

Parkinson's disease results from the gradual death of dopamine-producing cells in the brain. The brain functions like a factory with various neurotransmitters, and the deficiency of dopamine disrupts this factory's operations. This leads to Parkinson's symptoms such as slowness, tremors, and postural instability.

"Our brain isn't producing enough dopamine to function properly. What can we do?"
"The solution is to supply dopamine externally."

One might think consuming a lot of dopamine would solve the problem, but there's a catch. The brain is protected by the blood-brain barrier, a defense mechanism that prevents harmful substances from reaching the brain but also makes it difficult for beneficial substances to pass through. Dopamine is no exception.

Category	Chemical Name	Representative Drug Names
Levodopa	Levodopa	Sinemet, Madopar, Perkin, Myungdopar, Stalevo
Dopamine Agonists	Ropinirole, Pramipexole, Rotigotine	Requip, Mirapex, Neupro
Enzyme Inhibitors	MAO-B inhibitor, COMT inhibitor	Mao-B Tab, Azilect, Xadago, Comtan, etc.
Others	Anticholinergic	Amantadine, Trihexin

"How can we deliver dopamine to the brain?"

Significant research and effort have gone into this, and in 1968, a break-through was made with the development of Levodopa.

Levodopa can cross the blood-brain barrier and be converted into dopamine in the brain. Its introduction dramatically changed the lives of Parkinson's patients.

The movie "Awakenings," based on Oliver Sacks' work, illustrates how patients who were immobile for years began to move after taking Levodopa. It was a miraculous awakening.

Since the introduction of Levodopa, many medications for Parkinson's disease have been developed. Dopamine agonists are drugs that can act directly as dopamine in the brain without needing to go through the metabolic process. These drugs provide more consistent effects and have a longer duration of action compared to levodopa. However, their effectiveness may be somewhat less than that of levodopa. MAO-B inhibitors work by blocking the breakdown of dopamine, helping to keep it in the brain longer. The COMT inhibitor class of drugs also prevents the breakdown of dopamine. They help maintain higher levels of levodopa in the body by preventing its destruction. This is especially beneficial for Parkinson's patients who experience the "wearing-off" phenomenon, where the effects of levodopa diminish quickly.

Medication is fundamental and crucial in Parkinson's disease treatment. It's important to take the prescribed dosage consistently at scheduled times. Since symptoms and medication responses vary among individuals, it's necessary to adjust the dosage and type of medication in consultation with your doctor.

Most medications aim to alleviate Parkinson's symptoms rather than cure the disease. Like diabetes, which cannot be cured but can be managed with medication to control blood sugar levels and prevent complications, Parkinson's disease management focuses on symptom relief. Proper medication adherence is the first principle in treating Parkinson's disease.

5. LIMITATIONS OF PARKINSON'S MEDICATIONS

LONG-TERM SIDE EFFECTS OF PARKINSON'S MEDICATIONS

Levodopa is truly a life-changing medication for people with Parkinson's disease. Especially for those in the early stages, the effects of Levodopa can be remarkably positive. This period, when the medication works exceptionally well, is often referred to as the 'honeymoon period.' It's a time filled with hope and the belief that, with this drug, they can weather any storm. However, as time goes by, the sweet dream of this honeymoon phase inevitably begins to fade into reality. After about 4 to 5 years of long-term use, the limitations of Levodopa start to become apparent.

"In the early stages, a small dose of Levodopa greatly improved my symptoms. But over time, the effect diminished, and I needed higher doses and more medications."

The duration of the drug's effect shortens. Patients experience "off" periods (when the medication wears off) and "on" periods (when the medication is effective). Initially, one dose lasted all day, but eventually, the effect lasts only a few hours, causing difficulties between doses. This is known as the "wearing off" phenomenon, leading to more frequent dosing.

Motor fluctuations occur. It becomes extremely difficult to move when the medication's effect wears off, but after taking the medication, the body moves excessively on its own. This uncontrolled movement is called dyskinesia, which feels like the body is twisting and turning as if dancing, known as chorea. When the medication is active, dyskinesia occurs, and when the medication wears off, the body feels almost frozen.

Early in the morning, dystonia can also appear, causing the feet to curl inward and feel stiff.

As the disease progresses, medications may take longer to take effect ("delayed on"), and the transition between on and off periods becomes unpredictable. Sudden freezing episodes, where patients feel like they are stuck, can also happen.

Managing the side effects of Parkinson's medication involves adjusting the type, timing, and dosage of the drugs. Keeping a Parkinson's diary can be incredibly helpful in this process. In this diary, you should carefully note the names of the medications, the times you take them, and when you experience the "on" and "off" periods. This will help you understand how your body reacts to the medication. While you may not need to start keeping a Parkinson's diary from the very beginning, it becomes beneficial once you start feeling the effects of the medication wearing off. At this point, it would be wise to record your experiences and discuss them with your doctor during your outpatient visits.

Why Do Long-term Side Effects Occur?

These side effects commonly appear in mid-to-late-stage Parkinson's disease. They are not solely due to the medications but also reflect the progression of the disease, with fewer dopamine cells left to buffer changes.

A mountain full of sturdy trees will remain resilient despite changes in the weather. The early stages of Parkinson's disease are like that abundant mountain. The remaining dopamine nerve cells are relatively well-preserved. These nerve cells release dopamine steadily and consistently. When you take medication, the levodopa is absorbed, converted into dopamine, stored, and then slowly released. However, as the disease progresses, more degeneration occurs in the brain, and the number of functioning dopamine cells decreases. This leads to an unstable response to external medications. It becomes like a barren mountain with only a few trees left. A little rain can cause floods and landslides, but if it doesn't rain for a few days, a drought quickly sets in.

The textbook timeline for the appearance of drug side effects is typically stated as 3 to 5 years, but this can vary greatly depending on the patient. Based on personal experience, it seems that with recent improvements in medication and the increased knowledge and health of patients, many are able to manage their condition well with medication for more than five years. Meeting many wise patients who take good care of their medication and overall health gives me greater hope for the treatment of Parkinson's disease.

Should I Try to Manage Without Medication?

"I don't want to take Parkinson's medication."
"Why do you think that? Your symptoms suggest you need it."
"I'm afraid of the side effects. I heard they develop after five years. My symptoms are uncomfortable, but can I manage without medication for now?"

After taking medication for five years, side effects develop and the effectiveness wears off. So, would it be better to delay taking the medication as long as possible? This is a common question asked by Parkinson's patients worldwide in the clinic. Both patients and doctors are very curious about the answer to this question. About 20 years ago, there was a trend to delay using Levodopa as much as possible, using dopamine agonists as an alternative to manage the late-stage side effects of Levodopa. However, dopamine agonists alone did not produce satisfactory results. Additionally, in older patients, the side effects of dopamine agonists were significant. Research on Levodopa and its late-stage side effects has continued, and the latest findings conclude the following.

"It's not advisable to delay the use of levodopa due to concerns about late-stage side effects."

Here's a study that highlights this point.

An intriguing study conducted over four years in Italy and Ghana was published in the renowned journal "Brain" in 2014. The research compared two groups of Parkinson's patients: those in Ghana who, due to economic or medical reasons, couldn't take levodopa for several years and only started the medication when their condition worsened, and those in Italy who took levodopa as soon as they needed it. The question was whether the Ghanaian patients, who delayed levodopa use, experienced fewer late-stage motor complications than the Italian patients who took the medication earlier.

The study's conclusion was clear: delaying levodopa did not result in fewer late-stage motor complications. The factors that influenced these complications were the daily dose of levodopa and the duration of Parkinson's disease. In other words, the longer a person had Parkinson's, the more late-stage motor complications they experienced, and the higher the daily dose of levodopa, the more complications arose. The length of time a patient had been taking levodopa had no significant correlation with these side effects. Citing this research, Dr. Susan Fox and Dr. Anthony Lang advised on levodopa use:

"Don't delay, start today."

The goals of medication treatment for Parkinson's disease are threefold: symptom improvement, enhancement of quality of life, and increased survival rates. While medication primarily targets symptom management, it also significantly improves quality of life and increases the chances of survival. This has been proven through numerous studies. Therefore, medication treatment should not be seen as merely symptom relief, but as a critical approach to improving overall life quality and longevity for patients.

Don't hesitate to take medication because of misconceptions about long-term side effects. In fact, delaying medication can lead to a need for higher doses and more aggressive treatment to control symptoms, which in turn can increase the risk of side effects. Don't spend even one day struggling more than necessary. Taking medication appropriately, along with improving motor functions and leading a more active and fulfilling life, is the right approach to treatment.

Parkinson's Medications to be Cautious With

- Gastrointestinal Motility Drugs: Levosulpiride, Metoclopramide, Clebopride
- Antipsychotics: Haloperidol, Chlorpromazine, Fluphenazine, Promethazine, Prochlorperazine, Perphenazine, Pimozide, Sulpiride, Risperidone, Olanzapine, Ziprasidone, Aripiprazole
- Others: Flunarizine, Cinnarizine

There are times when taking the above medication is absolutely necessary. When you do need to take it, make sure to consult with a specialist and monitor any worsening of Parkinson's symptoms.

Seven Smart Tips for Taking Parkinson's Medication

"Are there things patients should be mindful of when taking their medication?"
"How can I manage my medication wisely and effectively?"

(1) Know Your Medications Well

Patients need to be fully aware of the medications they are taking. Different people react uniquely to specific medications, so it's crucial to keep a detailed record of what you're taking and how much. Make sure to note any side effects and remember them.

(2) Stick to Your Medication Schedule

Initially, you may not notice an immediate response to your medication. As the disease progresses, your response to medication may change. There are periods when the medication is effective (on-time) and periods when it isn't (off-time). It's important to take your medication at the same time each day to manage these cycles effectively.

(3) Maintain a Regular Eating Schedule

Inconsistent eating habits, like binge eating or skipping meals, can lead to irregular medication responses. Try to maintain a consistent eating schedule to help your medication work more reliably.

(4) Consult Your Doctor Before Making Changes

Some patients might adjust their medication on their own because they fear their doctor's reaction or disapproval. Don't do this. Always discuss your actual medication routine with your neurologist. They are there to help you and can provide the best advice.

(5) Report Side Effects to Your Doctor

Side effects can vary greatly from person to person. Share any sensations or information about adverse effects with your doctor so they can make necessary adjustments.

(6) Check Compatibility with Other Medications

It's common to be prescribed medications for other conditions besides Parkinson's. Always inform your doctor about your Parkinson's medications when you're prescribed new drugs. It's important to know if there are any interactions or conflicts with your Parkinson's medications.

(7) Don't Obsess Over Your Medication

While medication is crucial in managing Parkinson's, it's even more important to focus on yourself. What this means is, don't let your life revolve entirely around your illness and medication. It's not uncommon to see patients overly fixated on taking their meds perfectly on time or worrying excessively about dosages. Some read their medication guides repeatedly, trying to figure out the best approach. Remember, Parkinson's medication is there to supplement the dopamine your brain is lacking. Try not to stress too much about how the medication works or its side effects. Relax and take your medication calmly; this approach can help you feel more at ease both mentally and physically.

6. SURGICAL TREATMENT FOR PARKINSON'S DISEASE

The Story of Dopa Min, Considering Surgery

"Do they perform surgery for Parkinson's disease?"

Lately, I've been feeling very unsettled. Since last year, even though I've been taking my medication, it seems to be losing its effectiveness. My doctor increased the dosage, and while it definitely made moving easier, the effects didn't last long. Right before it's time for my next dose, my voice weakens, and I feel completely drained. We increased the frequency from three times a day to four, which helped a bit. But then something strange started happening. My arms and legs began moving on their own. Especially when the medication kicked in, my limbs would move too much. When I'm around others, I feel so embarrassed that I pretend to be doing exercises, flailing my arms and legs around.

My doctor tried various medications to observe these abnormal movements. There were slight improvements, but I was never completely satisfied. Having to take a handful of pills every hour is exhausting. My neurologist suggested something different.

"How about considering surgery?"

"Surgery? Do they perform surgery for Parkinson's disease?"

"Yes, there is a surgery called Deep Brain Stimulation (DBS). It involves placing an electrode in the part of the brain that controls movement. This electrode sends electrical impulses to help control Parkinson's symptoms."

"Oh, brain surgery? Does this mean Parkinson's disease can be cured?"

"DBS doesn't cure Parkinson's disease, but it can significantly improve motor function and quality of life. Many patients respond very well to it, and if your symptoms improve, you might be able to reduce your medication."

"Yes, but isn't brain surgery risky?"

"It is brain surgery, but it's not like the traditional kind where we open the brain completely. We only make a small hole for the electrode. There's about a 1-2% risk of complications like infection or brain hemorrhage. Other issues like inflammation or equipment problems can also occur. The surgery is usually done under anesthesia, but sometimes it's performed while the patient is awake."

Performing brain surgery on Parkinson's patients has been attempted for a long time. Before Levodopa was available, parts of the brain controlling tremors were destroyed to reduce dyskinesia. This method was invasive and had significant risks and side effects, so it was rarely done after medication was developed. However, since 1987, with the development of DBS, there have been remarkable improvements in symptoms, and many patients now benefit from this surgery. It has become a highly successful field in recent brain surgery advancements.

Dr. Alim-Louis Benabid in France first introduced DBS in 1987, and it was adopted in Korea in the 2000s. In 2004, it became covered by medical insurance, making it more widely available. DBS involves implanting a stimulator in the chest connected to electrodes in the brain that send electrical impulses.

The specific target areas for stimulation vary depending on the disease and symptoms, such as the globus pallidus, subthalamic nucleus, thalamus, and pedunculopontine nucleus. For Parkinson's disease, the subthalamic nucleus is the most common target. Recently, DBS targeting the pedunculopontine nucleus has shown good results in patients with gait disturbances. About 89-90% of patients have experienced significant improvements, with reduced dyskinesia and enhanced motor function. This also allowed for a reduction in medication, greatly improving their quality of life.

7. ARE YOU A CANDIDATE FOR SURGERY?

The effectiveness of DBS is clear, but not all patients are suitable candidates. About 15% of Parkinson's patients are considered eligible for this surgery. The criteria for determining eligibility are as follows:

(1) Confirmed Diagnosis of Idiopathic Parkinson's Disease for Over 5 Years

Parkinsonian syndromes and secondary Parkinsonism are not candidates for this surgery. Additionally, in the early stages after diagnosis, medication is prioritized over surgery. Surgery is considered only after at least 5 years have passed since diagnosis.

(2) Good Response to Levodopa

Patients who have responded well to Levodopa before surgery are likely to respond well to DBS. If medication has been ineffective, surgery is not recommended.

(3) Severe Motor Complications Despite Proper Medication

Patients who experience severe motor fluctuations or dyskinesia that significantly impair daily life despite appropriate medication may be candidates for surgery.

(4) Manageable Cognitive and Emotional Conditions

Cognitive and psychological assessments are performed. If dementia is suspected or if there is severe depression or anxiety, surgery is not recommended.

(5) Overall Good Health

Patients must be in good health otherwise, with no other conditions that would complicate brain surgery or worsen due to the surgery.

(6) Patients Under 75 Years Old

For elderly patients, there can be greater concern about surgical complications. It's known that younger patients tend to experience better improvements in motor function and respond more favorably to surgery. However, if an older patient is in good physical health, surgery can still be a viable option even if they are over 75 years old. In such cases, the outcomes can be significantly beneficial.

How Long Does Surgery's Effect Last?

Even after Deep Brain Stimulation (DBS) surgery, the patient's brain continues to age, and Parkinson's disease progresses. Naturally, one might wonder how long the effects of the surgery will last and how effective it will be compared to patients who do not undergo surgery. According to various studies, the effects of surgery, such as improved motor function, can last for one, two, or even five years post-surgery. This improvement is crucial as it directly impacts the quality of life. While not all patients are candidates for surgery, for those who are suitable, considering the surgery could be a beneficial choice.

8. OTHER TREATMENTS FOR PARKINSON'S DISEASE: EXERCISE AND REHABILITATION

Exercise and rehabilitation are critical for managing any illness, and this is especially true for Parkinson's disease, where motor symptoms progressively worsen. The treatment of Parkinson's disease can be divided into three main categories: medication, surgical treatment, and exercise therapy.

For Parkinson's patients, it is particularly important to maintain physical movement. Over time, joints can become stiff, and the range of motion decreases. Therefore engaging in regular exercise helps maintain maximum mobility and prevent muscle weakness.

Rehabilitation therapy from a specialized physical medicine department is highly recommended if accessible. For those experiencing balance issues or swallowing difficulties, working with skilled physical and occupational therapists can help improve balance and eating capabilities. The significance of exercise therapy will be further detailed in Chapters 3 and 4 of this book.

9. PARKINSON'S DISEASE AND REPETITIVE TRANSCRANIAL MAGNETIC STIMULATION (rTMS) THERAPY

I have a significant interest in Repetitive Transcranial Magnetic Stimulation (rTMS) therapy. Operating a neurology clinic, I have set up a TMS treatment facility.

rTMS involves using a powerful magnetic field generated by an electromagnetic coil to pass through the skull and either activate or inhibit specific neurons in the brain. This technique is FDA-approved in the United States for treating depression, headaches, and obsessive-compulsive disorder, and it is applied to many neurological conditions worldwide. The procedure does not require anesthesia and has minimal side effects. Patients receive brain stimulation in a seated position for about 20-30 minutes, making it a very convenient treatment.

For over 20 years, research on the treatment of Parkinson's disease using rTMS has been actively ongoing. It's important to note that rTMS is not a replacement for medication or deep brain stimulation (DBS). Unlike DBS, rTMS cannot provide continuous stimulation deep within the brain. However, one of the significant advantages of rTMS is that it is non-invasive, meaning it does not require brain surgery like DBS does. By transmitting magnetic waves to the brain, rTMS aims to alter the excitability of nerve cells, which can help alleviate the symptoms of Parkinson's disease.

In 2006, a significant study on the effects of rTMS on Parkinson's disease was published. Dr. Mikhail Lomarev's team conducted a double-blind placebo-controlled study on 18 Parkinson's patients, examining the effects of rTMS on gait and bradykinesia. Patients were divided into real and sham rTMS groups. Over four weeks, they completed eight rTMS sessions and underwent motor function assessments before and after treatment. Those in the real rTMS group showed significant improvements in walking speed and hand motor skills compared to the sham group, with effects lasting for a month after treatment.

Subsequent studies produced varying results. In 2015, a large-scale analysis of 20 studies involving 470 subjects concluded that high-frequency rTMS of the motor cortex or low-frequency rTMS of the frontal lobe effectively improved motor symptoms in Parkinson's patients. Research continues to refine the optimal protocols, focusing on stimulation frequency, location, and symptom types. Recently, Dr. Wenjie Zhang's team published a comprehensive analysis of research findings from 1988 to 2022. Notably, they consistently reported that high-frequency stimulation of both motor cortices had a positive effect on motor symptoms, such as freezing of gait and the motor section of the Unified Parkinson's Disease Rating Scale (UPDRS Part III).

rTMS is also effective in treating depression in Parkinson's patients. Stimulating the left dorsolateral prefrontal cortex (DLPFC) showed improvement in depression after 10 sessions, with effects lasting up to five weeks. Based on this evidence, the 2020 Clinical Neurophysiology Society guidelines rated rTMS as a high-evidence treatment for depression in Parkinson's patients.

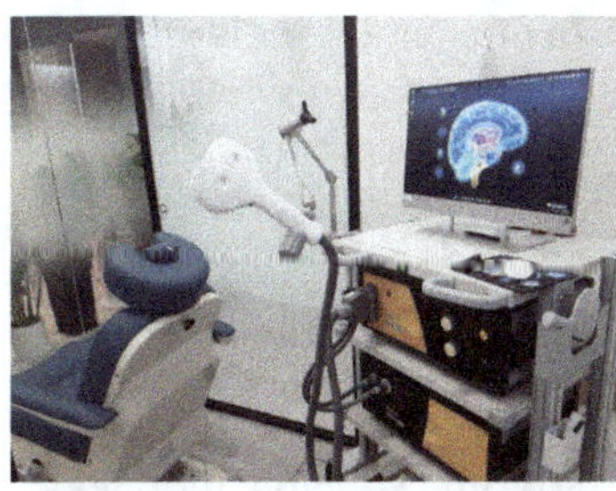

Transcranial Magnetic Stimulation Treatment Room at Brainup Neurology Clinic

Although rTMS is gaining attention as a non-invasive brain stimulation treatment, more research is needed to map the most effective brain regions, stimulation protocols, and parameters for treating Parkinson's disease. What is clear is that rTMS positively impacts neuroplasticity and is expected to play an expanding role in motor control and brain function activation.

10. THE PROGRESSION OF PARKINSON'S DISEASE

WHAT STAGE OF PARKINSON'S DISEASE AM I IN?

"Parkinson's disease is said to be a progressive condition, so how far along am I?"
"Does Parkinson's disease have stages like cancer does?"

Parkinson's disease, like other degenerative diseases, progresses over time. It is categorized into five stages based on motor symptoms, known as the Hoehn and Yahr stages:

Stage 1: Symptoms are limited to one side of the body.
Stage 2: Symptoms appear on both sides but do not impair balance.
Stage 3: Symptoms on both sides, with impaired balance and walking difficulty.
Stage 4: Severe symptoms but still able to walk independently.
Stage 5: Unable to walk independently, requiring a wheelchair or being bedridden.

James Park: His right hand trembles, and its movement feels weak. Occasionally, his right leg also trembles and slows down when walking. However, his left side is unaffected, and he maintains good balance without swallowing difficulties. Mr. Park is in Hoehn and Yahr Stage 1.

Dopa Min: Her movements in both arms and legs are significantly impaired. Especially when the medication wears off, it's extremely difficult for her to move. She can barely get up to go to the bathroom. She wobbles, looking like she might fall, and has a hard time keeping her balance. Although she can still manage on her own, it's really tough. Dopa Min is at stage 4 on the Hoehn and Yahr scale.

However, about 20 minutes after taking her medication, Dopa Min gains a fair amount of strength. While her arm and leg movements are not as good as those of a healthy person, they become much lighter. She wobbles less and feels less like she might fall. During this time when the medication is effective, she can, albeit slowly, manage some household chores. When the medication is working, Dopa Min is at stage 3 on the Hoehn and Yahr scale.

The stages of Parkinson's disease refer to the severity of motor symptoms. Unlike cancer, a higher stage does not mean the patient will not respond to medication. For example, a patient who is at stage 4 may improve to stage 2 or 3 after taking medication.

What's important in stages 2 and 3 is the sense of balance. In stage 2, the patient can maintain balance well, but if their sense of balance starts to decline, they are considered to have entered stage 3. The Hoehn and Yahr scale is widely used clinically, and it also helps in planning future exercise routines based on the stage. Knowing which stage you are in can be very helpful.

PART 3.
PARKINSON'S DISEASE AND EXERCISE

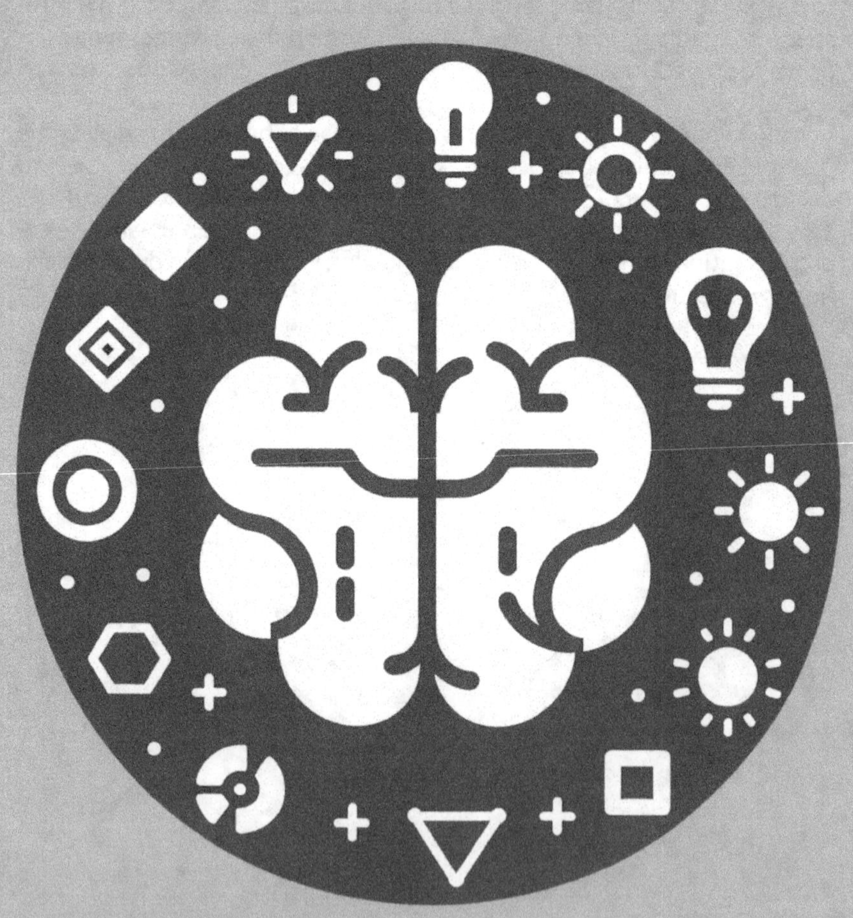

1. THE IMPORTANCE OF EXERCISE THERAPY

James Park's Exercise Journey

It's been about six months since I was diagnosed with Parkinson's disease and started taking medication. Now, I truly feel like I'm living as a Parkinson's patient. My symptoms haven't worsened, and it seems like the medication is helping.

"Hello, Mr. Park. How are you today?"
"No particular discomfort, it seems. Are you keeping up with your exercise?"

The doctor greets me warmly, as always. Every doctor and every book and video about Parkinson's disease always emphasize the importance of exercise. I know exercise is supposed to be good for me, but I'm not exactly sure what kind of exercise or how to do it properly. Honestly, I'm not even convinced that exercise is essential for Parkinson's disease. So, I decided to ask a tricky question.

"Every time I come to the hospital, the doctor always talks about 'exercise.' But I'm skeptical. Whether it's diabetes, high blood pressure, or cancer, everyone just says exercise is good for health, right? So, is exercise just a nice thing to do for Parkinson's, or does it really have a significant impact?"

"Exercise has been scientifically proven to be beneficial for Parkinson's disease through numerous research papers. Exercise offers several benefits for Parkinson's patients. It can alleviate the symptoms of Parkinson's disease, improve brain plasticity, and provide

> social and emotional benefits that are very positive for managing Parkinson's."
>
> Hearing a medical explanation like this makes me want to study exercise therapy more deeply. I've lived my life as a researcher, so this habit of delving deep into topics doesn't fade, even with Parkinson's disease.

Does Exercise Really Help with Parkinson's Disease?

Treatment for Parkinson's disease can be divided into three main categories: medication, surgical treatment, and exercise therapy. Medications need to be taken diligently every day, with close monitoring of their effects and side effects. When considering surgery, patients encounter a lot of research, discussions, and advice before making a decision. Exercise is listed as a treatment in almost every textbook, but its importance often seems undervalued. Does exercise really make a difference in Parkinson's disease? Like Mr. Park's question, is it just common sense that exercise is good, or is there more to it?

In this chapter, we will take a more scientific approach to understanding the role of exercise in Parkinson's disease. Modern medicine is "evidence-based." To say that something is effective, there must be substantial evidence. Medications for Parkinson's disease have undergone clinical trials to prove their efficacy. These studies compare the effects and side effects of the drug in groups who take the medication versus those who do not. The same principle applies to exercise. Many studies have been conducted to prove that exercise is effective for Parkinson's disease. Fortunately, the results show that exercise has very positive effects on Parkinson's.

We will analyze exercise from an evidence-based medicine perspective, using research and papers from various centers around the world to explain its benefits. If you find this section too difficult to read, feel free to skip to Chapter 4. To summarize Chapter 3, "Exercise is very important in Parkinson's disease."

2. THE BENEFITS OF EXERCISE FOR PARKINSON'S DISEASE

First, let's define "physical activity" and "exercise."

"Physical activity" is a broad term that includes any movement of our muscles that uses energy. This can include work tasks, household chores, hobbies, cycling, cleaning, and organizing. In daily life, we tend to conserve energy and try to make tasks less strenuous. Among various physical activities is exercise, which is deliberately structured to consume more energy. Exercise is planned, structured, and repetitive physical activity aimed at improving overall health.

In the context of treatment, terms like "exercise therapy," "physical activity therapy," "rehabilitation therapy," and "occupational therapy" are used, each with slight differences in meaning. While "exercise" and "physical activity" are distinct terms, we will use them interchangeably in this book for simplicity. For ease of understanding, we will use "exercise therapy" to refer to all therapies related to physical activity.

Recent research on exercise therapy for Parkinson's disease is very active. There are numerous studies and large-scale meta-analyses, Cochrane reviews, and prospective studies being published. Exercise helps release neuroprotective substances in the brain, increases oxygenation, and promotes the growth of new cells and longevity. Specifically, exercise benefits Parkinson's disease in three major ways.

First, it alleviates Parkinson's symptoms.

Second, it slows the progression of the disease.

Third, it improves quality of life and reinforces the value of being a social human being.

3. EXERCISE IMPROVES PARKINSON'S SYMPTOMS

Dr. Tomlinson's team in the UK reviewed existing studies on exercise therapy for Parkinson's disease. They compared groups who participated in exercise therapy to those who did not, highlighting the benefits of exercise. The study included 39 studies with a total of 1,827 participants. They compared walking speed, freezing of gait, stride length, falls, balance, and the Unified Parkinson's Disease Rating Scale (UPDRS). The results showed that patients in the exercise therapy group performed better.

Parkinson's disease manifests as movement symptoms that make it difficult to move. Along with changes in movement itself, there are gradual changes in how our brain perceives movement. Compared to healthy adults, Parkinson's patients have weaker muscle strength and intensity, leading to slower walking speed, balance issues, and a higher risk of falling. Exercise helps maintain balance, makes movement easier, and improves daily activities. It also strengthens muscles, improves walking, and helps prevent falls.

Parkinson's patients experience slower and smaller movements. Actions like bending over or walking become smaller, a condition known as hypokinesia. When walking, they take short, shuffling steps and swing their arms less. Handwriting becomes smaller, and their voice may become softer. The brain adjusts to perceive these smaller movements as normal. Exercise therapy helps expand the range of motion in daily activities. It uses muscles that aren't used much and promotes diverse and large movements of the joints. Exercise intentionally trains larger movements.

Exercise increases calcium levels in the blood, which is then transported to the brain. This enhances the dopamine production process through the calmodulin-dependent system. Increased dopamine levels make various brain functions more flexible. In laboratory studies, epileptic and hypertensive rats with very low dopamine levels in the neostriatum and nucleus accumbens showed significant improvement in dopamine levels after exercise training. It's believed that exercise positively influences the calcium/calmodulin-dependent dopamine formation process, increasing dopamine levels. This suggests that for Parkinson's disease and even age-related dementia, exercise-induced dopamine increase can significantly improve symptoms.

Furthermore exercise helps correct postural deformities, stretches muscles and joints, and aids in recovering flexibility. As the disease progresses, muscles become stiff, and joint rigidity is observed. Flexibility decreases, and posture becomes stooped, often accompanied by pain. Exercise strengthens core muscles and promotes an upright posture. Additionally, strengthening muscles enhances quickness and balance, reducing the likelihood of falls. Thus, exercise has a direct alleviating effect on Parkinson's symptoms.

4. EXERCISE DELAYS DEMENTIA

Parkinson's disease leads to the death of brain cells, with the affected area gradually expanding. This results in non-motor symptoms in addition to the typical motor symptoms of Parkinson's disease, with cognitive decline, such as dementia, being a significant concern. Exercise also has a positive impact on cognitive function. Notable studies have shown that along with slowing the progression of Parkinson's motor symptoms, exercise also reduces cognitive decline.

A recent study analyzed the impact of exercise on the cognitive function of Parkinson's patients over the past decade. This analysis included nine studies that tracked the cognitive abilities of patients who exercised compared to those who did not. Cognitive function can be categorized into various aspects such as memory, visuospatial abilities, executive function, attention, and frontal lobe function. Dementia in Parkinson's patients is particularly known to affect frontal lobe function and executive function more severely. The study found that regardless of the type of exercise—whether dance, treadmill training, or combined exercises—Parkinson's patients who exercised scored higher on cognitive function tests.

Exercise was especially beneficial in improving executive function and frontal lobe function.

Executive function and frontal lobe function are akin to the steering wheel of our thoughts. When we aim to reach a destination, we press the accelerator to speed up. If a red light appears, we immediately hit the brakes. If a roadblock suddenly appears in our path, we quickly find an alternate route to reach our goal. Executive function is the brain's ability to plan and execute tasks to achieve a specific goal. It also allows us to swiftly switch settings in our brain to take a different path when necessary.

The frontal lobe, in particular, plays a crucial role in applying the brakes when needed. It regulates our impulses, such as appetite and sexual desire, ensuring that we don't act solely on our urges. Therefore, people with well-developed frontal lobe functions tend to have admirable social qualities. When you see a child throwing a tantrum in a store because they didn't get a toy, think, "Ah, their frontal lobe hasn't fully developed yet. I hope their frontal lobe matures well."

In Parkinson's disease, it's not just the decline in cognitive function that patients have to contend with. Many non-motor symptoms also arise, such as sleep disturbances, depression, and autonomic nervous system issues like constipation or dizziness. These non-motor symptoms are major factors that reduce the quality of life for patients. It's easy to understand that exercise, which involves physical movement, can improve the motor symptoms of Parkinson's disease. Furthermore, what is even more impressive is that exercise significantly improves these non-motor symptoms as well. Patients experience better sleep, reduced depression and chronic fatigue, and enhanced concentration and cognitive function, all of which lead to an overall improvement in their quality of life.

One study objectively measured changes in sleep quality rather than relying on subjective feelings. This study involved Parkinson's patients over the age of 45 in the Hoehn and Yahr stages 2-3. The participants were divided into two groups: one that exercised three times a week for 16 weeks and one that did not exercise. Sleep quality was assessed at the beginning and end of the study using polysomnography.

The results were striking. The group that engaged in high-intensity exercise experienced overall improvements in sleep. They fell asleep faster, had longer total sleep times, and most importantly, increased the amount of deep sleep. The effects of exercise were immediate and profound, making it highly recommended for anyone struggling with insomnia.

5. EXERCISE SLOWS THE PROGRESSION OF PARKINSON'S DISEASE

Parkinson's disease progresses slowly. It occurs because brain cells gradually die off. Wouldn't it be wonderful if we could stop this progression or at least slow it down? If there were a treatment that could prevent brain cells from dying, our brains wouldn't age anymore. It would be like finding the elixir of youth. The ultimate goal in treating Parkinson's disease is to slow its progression. It's not just about managing the symptoms but about slowing down or halting the disease itself. This is known as disease modification.

There is an old house. Over the years, its windows have broken, and it's falling apart in various places. Summer and fall were bearable, but once winter hits, the house becomes unbearably cold. What should we do? We try putting on thick coats, wearing hats, and gloves. We even light a fire in the hearth with some logs. These measures help us endure the cold for now. This is like symptomatic treatment.

But what would be a more fundamental solution? It would be fixing the broken windows. We also need to replace the loose door and properly insulate the walls. We seal up every gap where the harsh winter wind can seep through. These actions represent more fundamental treatments, which is what we mean by 'disease modification.'

Exercise has been shown to slow the progression of Parkinson's and protect brain cells. In 2019, Dr. Paul and his team studied the impact of exercise on the progression of Parkinson's disease. They analyzed 244 patients who had been diagnosed with Parkinson's for less than three years. The study examined their participation in competitive sports and their overall physical activity levels. Five years later, they found that patients with higher physical activity levels experienced slower disease progression.

Similar results were found in the National Parkinson's Foundation Quality Improvement Initiative (NPF-QII), which included 4,866 participants. They divided participants into three groups based on their weekly exercise levels and observed Parkinson's progression after one year. Those who engaged in "regular exercise" for more than two and a half hours per week showed significantly better motor symptoms compared to those who exercised less or not at all.

One notable study among Parkinson's patient research cohorts is the PPMI (Parkinson's Progressive Markers Initiative) study. This study investigated the relationship between physical activity levels in older adults and the progression of Parkinson's disease. It found that higher levels of physical activity were associated with slower progression of Parkinson's disease over a two-year period. This indicates that exercise not only has a positive effect on the symptoms of Parkinson's disease but also offers protective benefits against neurodegeneration.

Animal studies have delved deeper into the fundamental effects of exercise on the brain. These studies revealed that exercise promotes the secretion of neurotrophic growth factors, which have neuroprotective functions. Exercise stimulates the expression of substances like GDNF (glia cell-derived neurotrophic factor) and BDNF (brain-derived neurotrophic factor), which help combat neurotoxic substances. Additionally, exercise has antioxidant and anti-inflammatory effects, playing a beneficial role in counteracting oxidative stress, mitochondrial dysfunction, and neuroinflammation—all of which contribute to the death of brain nerve cells.

These changes in the brain from exercising are like repairing broken windows and sealing up holes to withstand the harsh winter wind. Ideally, we'd tear down the house and rebuild it from scratch, but we can't turn back time or become young again. However, we can remodel how our bodies and brains function through exercise. Exercise is an incredibly valuable therapy.

6. EXERCISE AS A SOURCE OF SOCIAL VALUE

Humans are social animals, and we find happiness living together. Recently, our lives have trended towards 'contactless' interactions. Many people find it easier to do things alone and avoid meeting others. Yet, even those who eat alone constantly engage with others through their smartphones. While avoiding face-to-face interactions might reduce emotional stress, people still form clubs and groups with like-minded individuals. They find comfort in online communities where they can connect with others who share similar interests. Despite changes in how we interact, the need to connect with others for stability and happiness remains constant.

Parkinson's patients often find their social circles shrinking after diagnosis. Due to physical discomfort, they may avoid gatherings. More often, it's the psychological impact that makes them withdraw from social activities. If being part of a gathering is uncomfortable and stressful, it's understandable not to want to spend energy on it. However, social interaction is essential. Exercise can provide new opportunities to meet people. Even if you're not exercising with like-minded individuals, simply greeting and chatting with people you encounter can be a positive experience.

Exercise fosters a positive mindset and boosts confidence. Gradually expand your activity range through exercise. Social gatherings that once felt daunting may become more approachable. Additionally, as movement becomes easier with exercise, you'll find more time and energy for social activities. Don't underestimate your physical abilities. Avoid prematurely deciding something is impossible; instead, find the strength to challenge yourself.

Patients in the later stages of Parkinson's have fewer opportunities for social interaction and thus meet fewer people. Some may be confined to their beds in hospitals. For these individuals, help with physical activities and exercise is crucial. Relationships and time spent with those who assist with exercise are excellent opportunities to prevent social isolation. One study analyzed the improved quality of life in a group that participated in exercise. The benefits were attributed not only to the exercise itself but also to the emotional connections formed with therapists and others during the program. The value of being socially engaged can be extended and deepened through exercise.

7. CAN EXERCISE PREVENT PARKINSON'S DISEASE?

Exercise as a Predictor of Parkinson's Disease: James Park's Story

Reading various research papers, I logically understood that exercise significantly benefits Parkinson's disease. Reflecting on my busy life and how I often neglected exercise, I wonder if my lack of physical activity led to my Parkinson's diagnosis. Today, I must ask this question during my appointment.

"Hello, Professor. I found the papers you sent on exercise fascinating. I have one more question. Did I get Parkinson's because I neglected exercise? Or does regular exercise reduce the risk of Parkinson's?"

"Hello. It's impressive that you read all those papers, and I'm glad you found them interesting. To summarize your question, exercise can be considered a predictive factor for Parkinson's disease."

"A predictive factor?"

"Yes, conditions that may reduce the likelihood of developing Parkinson's. For example, does exercising regularly lower the risk of Parkinson's? Similarly, a 'risk factor' is something that increases the likelihood of a disease. Like smoking is known to increase the risk of lung cancer, smoking is a risk factor for lung cancer."

Risk Factors for Parkinson's Disease

How can we avoid getting Parkinson's disease? This is a common question when faced with the disease. The cause of Parkinson's lies in the gradual death of dopamine-related brain cells. But among billions of people, why did I get Parkinson's? There's no straightforward answer. Essentially, we don't know. Heavy smoking increases the risk of lung disease, and daily alcohol consumption can damage the liver. However, it's hard to pinpoint specific behaviors that cause Parkinson's. Still, we wonder if there are factors that made us more susceptible.

The causes can be divided into two main categories: 'genetic factors' and 'environmental factors.' There are cases of Parkinson's caused by genetic abnormalities. Several genes are involved. In fact, genetic testing for Parkinson's is available in hospitals. But most Parkinson's cases, especially those occurring with age, rarely involve genetic abnormalities. Advances in genetics and computing have allowed detailed analysis of human genes, creating genetic maps. Hopefully, in the near future, we will understand which genetic functions lead to Parkinson's, revealing more about its origins.

Except for those born with genes predisposing them to Parkinson's, it's challenging to determine why the disease develops. There's a field of study that investigates why some people get certain diseases less frequently than others. This is called epidemiology. It involves long-term tracking of large groups of people, studying their habits, environment, genetic factors, and disease causation. Particularly with degenerative diseases, identifying these relationships is extremely challenging.

Epidemiological studies come in various forms. The study groups are called 'cohorts.' There are cohorts of people with specific diseases and cohorts from local communities.

One type of community-based cohort study involves observing a large group of ordinary people over an extended period. Researchers gather data on their height, weight, blood tests, cognitive function, and lifestyle habits such as coffee consumption, alcohol, smoking, exercise, and diet. They also collect information on family relationships, education, occupation, personality, and social interactions. This process gathers vast amounts of data. By tracking which diseases develop over the years, researchers analyze correlations with numerous factors. The outcomes can be unpredictable, and the causal relationships may not be clear.

Moreover, tracking large groups for extended periods makes such epidemiological studies very challenging. There are epidemiological studies related to Parkinson's disease, just like for other conditions. These studies analyze risk factors to determine which tendencies might make someone more susceptible to Parkinson's. According to various studies, though the results differ, it seems that people who consume coffee, drink alcohol in moderation, or smoke cigarettes might have a lower risk of developing Parkinson's.

Wait, what? Smoking cigarettes lowers the risk of Parkinson's disease? I can almost see the smiles on smokers' faces. But let's be clear: smoking significantly increases the risk of lung disease and various cancers. It also lowers life expectancy, meaning you might die much earlier, possibly before developing Parkinson's. So, please don't use the slim chance of reduced Parkinson's risk as an excuse to keep smoking. I strongly urge you to quit.

How about exercise? Do people who regularly exercise have a lower risk of developing Parkinson's? There are epidemiological studies on this too. Some studies suggest no correlation between exercise and Parkinson's incidence, while others indicate that exercise might reduce the risk.

Let's look at a large cohort study conducted in Sweden. This study included a whopping 43,368 participants and tracked them for 12.6 years to study the incidence of Parkinson's disease. The group that engaged in a lot of physical activity, whether through household chores or work, had a lower incidence of Parkinson's compared to the less active group. Interestingly, this effect was more pronounced in men, while there was no significant correlation in women.

Professor Chen's group also researched the relationship between physical activity and Parkinson's disease. They studied 48,574 men in the Health Professionals Follow-Up Study (HPFS) and 77,254 women in the

Nurses' Health Study (NHS). In the male group, the 30% with the highest level of physical activity had about a 30% lower incidence of Parkinson's compared to the least active group. However, in this cohort too, there was no significant correlation between physical activity and Parkinson's incidence in women.

With each study using different methodologies and producing varying results, it can be confusing to determine whether exercise truly lowers the risk of Parkinson's or not. However, large scale meta-analyses have consistently found a strong correlation between reduced Parkinson's risk and factors like smoking and coffee consumption. Although exercise might not show as strong a correlation as smoking and coffee, many studies still suggest that it benefits Parkinson's prevention. Moreover, physical activity and exercise are known to reduce the incidence of various cardiovascular and age-related degenerative diseases.

Are you worried about getting Parkinson's? This is a common question for children of parents with Parkinson's disease. What can you do to prevent it?

There is a clear answer. Increase the amount of physical activity in your daily life and make exercise a habit. Regular exercise and healthy lifestyle habits, along with drinking plenty of tea, can be very beneficial.

8. EFFECTIVE EXERCISES FOR PARKINSON'S DISEASE

James Park's Story

"There are so many types of exercise. What exercises are best for Parkinson's disease?"

"Many people ask this question. If you asked Parkinson's experts worldwide, they would all give the same answer."

All the experts agree? Now I'm really curious about what the best exercise for Parkinson's is.

"The best exercise for Parkinson's disease is any exercise you can do safely, regularly, and enjoyably."

"That answer is a bit disappointing. Isn't there any specific exercise that's particularly good for Parkinson's? I'm really curious."

Effective Exercises for Parkinson's Disease

This is a question that not only patients but also doctors and researchers are curious about.

"What exercises are good for Parkinson's disease?"

Researchers have analyzed and tested various forms of exercise to determine which ones are effective for Parkinson's. These include tango, treadmill running, resistance training (strength training), tai chi, qigong, boxing, aquatic therapy, dances like the waltz and foxtrot, yoga, mixed exercise programs, cycling, and Wii Fit. Let's look at the results from 106 physical activity studies conducted between 1981 and 2015. Fortunately, most forms of exercise significantly improved various exercise capacity indices, regardless of the type of exercise. Additionally, exercise in any form positively impacts mental symptoms, improving sleep, maintaining a happier and clearer mind, and giving a sense of purpose in life.

The key to exercise therapy is simply 'doing it.' So, the best exercise for you is the one you enjoy. Enjoyment makes you more likely to stick with it, and consistency leads to better treatment outcomes. Whether it's dancing, practicing yoga, walking in the pool, or strolling around your neighborhood, it all counts. You don't need to stick to just one activity. One day you can focus on intense training at the gym, the next day you might walk along a river, and another day you can ride a stationary bike at home. Increasing physical activity, even outside of formal exercise routines, is a positive lifestyle change. The first step in exercise therapy is to spend more time moving your body and working up a sweat.

If you want to be more systematic about your favorite exercises, try incorporating these four types of activities:

First, Resistance and Flexibility Exercises
Second, Aerobic Exercises
Third, Balance Exercises
Forth, Speech and Swallowing Exercises

Aerobic exercises include walking, climbing stairs, riding a stationary bike, and walking in a swimming pool. These exercises form the foundation and significantly improve cardiovascular health and overall fitness. Resistance exercises focus on building muscle strength, especially in the lower body. For people with Parkinson's, it's crucial to pair strength training with thorough stretching to maintain joint flexibility. Balance exercises are also important. The type of exercise can vary greatly depending on the stage of Parkinson's disease. For issues like choking or a soft voice, exercises such as speaking loudly, swallowing training, and singing are beneficial. All these exercises are interconnected. For instance, strength training combined with flexibility exercises can improve balance and walking. Examples of exercises will be detailed in Chapter 4. Dancing is an excellent form of exercise. It's enjoyable and engaging. The music provides auditory stimulation, and the dance movements ensure full joint movement. If dancing feels too challenging, start by moving slowly to music. Let the music guide you, and you might find a smile naturally appearing on your face.

9. HOW MUCH EXERCISE IS ENOUGH?

The World Health Organization (WHO) recommends the following for those aged 65 and older:

"Engage in at least 150 minutes of moderate-intensity aerobic exercise per week, or at least 75 minutes of vigorous-intensity aerobic physical activity."

Examples of moderate-intensity aerobic exercises include brisk walking at 3 to 4 miles per hour, cycling less than 10 miles per hour, or playing doubles tennis. Vigorous-intensity exercises include running, swimming laps, hiking, or cycling at more than 10 miles per hour. (American Heart Association)

Are we meeting these standards? About 33% of adults worldwide fall short of these guidelines. Unfortunately, people with Parkinson's disease tend to exercise even less. Only one-third of Parkinson's patients manage to walk for 30 minutes a day. A survey of 4,866 early-stage Parkinson's patients found that more than half exercised less than an hour and a half per week or didn't exercise at all. Given that Parkinson's disease progressively impairs movement, it's understandable that physical activity can be challenging. However, this makes securing exercise time even more crucial.

Exercise Three Times a Week for at Least 30 Minutes

Early-stage Parkinson's patients often don't feel significantly impaired and may neglect exercise. Those in mid-stage or beyond may feel discouraged by their decreased physical abilities and fear starting exercise. Regardless of your current situation, it's essential to extend your physical activity. Aim for at least an hour and a half of exercise per week. This is the minimum. Ideally, exercise for at least 30 minutes, three times a week. The exercise should be intense enough to get your heart rate up, equivalent to walking three miles in an hour.

Parkinson's disease is characterized by a gradual decrease in physical activity. This reduction happens faster and more severely in people with Parkinson's compared to the general population. Therefore, it's vital for those with Parkinson's to actively monitor and ensure they're getting enough exercise and physical activity.

10. THE FIVE PRINCIPLES OF BRAIN-ENHANCING EXERCISE

1. High-Intensity Activity Maximizes Neural Interactions
2. Complex Activities Are Better Than Simple Ones
3. Reward Yourself—Activities with Rewards Boost Dopamine Levels
4. Dopamine Neurons Respond to Movement—Use it, or lose it!
5. Start Early to Slow the Progression of Parkinson's

Dr. Fox and his team propose these five principles to enhance neural plasticity in Parkinson's patients. Neural plasticity, a somewhat complex concept, can be simply understood as the nervous system's ability to change itself. The term plasticity comes from the Latin word "plasticus," meaning "capable of being molded."

Imagine you sculpt a beautiful giraffe out of clay, but then your younger sibling runs in, snaps the giraffe's neck, and runs off. Frustrated, you mold the clay back together, but the dried parts make the giraffe's neck shorter, turning it into something that looks more like a horse. If the clay had completely dried and hardened, it would have been much harder to repair. However, since it was still pliable, you could reshape it. This flexibility is what we mean by plasticity. Neural plasticity refers to the nervous system's ability to adapt functionally and structurally in response to experience or injury. It's essential for adapting to aging, environmental changes, and diseases. The greater the neural plasticity, the better the brain can adapt to damage.

Exercise is one of the most effective ways to enhance neural plasticity in the brain of a Parkinson's patient. It can bring about significant changes in a brain where dopamine neurons are dying.

To maximize the benefits of exercise on neural plasticity, let's follow Dr. Fox's advice:

1. High-Intensity Exercise: Engaging in vigorous exercise, as opposed to light or moderate activities, increases interactions between brain cells.
2. Complex Activities: Complex exercises that require more coordination and thought stimulate structural adaptations in brain cells better than simple, repetitive activities.
3. Rewards: Winning a game or receiving any reward for exercise increases dopamine levels in the brain, enhancing learning and relearning processes.
4. Movement and Dopamine Neurons: Dopamine neurons are highly responsive to movement. Exercise them, or they will deteriorate from inactivity.
5. Start Now: Begin exercising early in the disease to slow its progression.

In the context of Parkinson's, exercise is like Merlin training young Arthur. Before meeting Merlin, Arthur was just a simple squire, unaware of his true potential. Merlin saw something special in Arthur and decided to mentor him. Arthur himself didn't change—his genes and brain cells were the same. But through Merlin's teachings and guidance, Arthur's brain cells became more active, interacting more and shining brightly. Despite his noble lineage, he couldn't realize his destiny until Merlin's training awakened his dormant abilities. His once inactive brain became vibrant and active. Without Merlin's guidance, Arthur would have remained an ordinary squire, never becoming the legendary King Arthur.

Parkinson's disease and other degenerative conditions involve the gradual death of brain cells. If you don't use these cells, they will continue to die. But if you nurture and use them, the remaining neurons will start working. For us, exercise is our Merlin.

The Five Principles of Exercise to Awaken Your Brain

Work Hard: Engage in vigorous exercise.

Do Complex Exercises: Incorporate activities that require coordination and thought.

Reward Yourself: Celebrate your achievements and progress.

Move to Keep Your Brain Alive: Exercise keeps your brain active; inactivity leads to deterioration.

Start Early: Begin exercising as soon as possible to slow disease progression.

11. GOALS OF REHABILITATION THERAPY

The primary treatment for Parkinson's disease is medication. However, exercise is also crucial. If you want to learn more about exercise therapy, it is beneficial to seek help from a rehabilitation medicine specialist. European clinical guidelines outline the general goals of rehabilitation for Parkinson's disease patients. The aim of rehabilitation therapy is to optimize the patient's activity, participation, and quality of life by considering individual functional and environmental factors. Rehabilitation therapy helps patients understand their physical capabilities and environmental factors, maximizing their ability to manage daily life effectively.

When you visit a rehabilitation medicine clinic, your condition will be assessed, and treatment tailored to your needs will begin. Neurodevelopmental treatment (NDT) involves one-on-one training with a skilled therapist. If you experience weakness or reduced motor skills on one side of your body, you will engage in strength training exercises. For those with gait disturbances, walking training is conducted with a therapist. Exercises to improve balance are also included. If assistive devices are needed, you will learn how to use them and incorporate them into your daily life. The training is customized to each person, which is its greatest advantage, as it addresses individual deficiencies. In addition to one-on-one neurodevelopmental therapy, group aerobic exercises are also conducted.

Another important aspect of rehabilitation therapy is occupational therapy. In occupational therapy, you practice movements needed for daily living. For example, if fine motor skills make using chopsticks difficult, you will train to improve these skills. Cognitive training is also provided through board games and role-playing activities. This, too, is tailored to individual needs. Swallowing rehabilitation is included, as Parkinson's disease can cause dysphagia, leading to frequent choking while eating. Training is provided to improve swallowing abilities and reduce the risk of aspiration. Speech therapy is also part of rehabilitation, addressing issues like reduced voice volume and unclear pronunciation to enhance communication abilities. Rehabilitation therapy thus covers all aspects of life, from motor skills to daily living abilities, making it a comprehensive treatment. It is also meticulously personalized.

The "Expert Consensus Recommendations for Rehabilitation Therapy for Parkinson's Disease Patients" published by the Korean Society for NeuroRehabilitation in 2020 outlines the goals of rehabilitation therapy for Parkinson's disease. A thorough understanding of the diagnosis and progression stage of Parkinson's disease is required to set personalized rehabilitation therapy goals.

Rehabilitation therapy can be described as "seeing the forest while looking at the trees." It not only focuses on each uncomfortable movement but also considers the patient's occupation, social conditions, and home environment to improve their quality of life. I hope many people will visit the rehabilitation medicine clinic and continue with consistent rehabilitation therapy.

"When is the best time to visit the rehabilitation medicine clinic?"
"When should rehabilitation therapy start, and how long should it continue?"

The best time to visit is immediately after diagnosis. However, in the very early stages of diagnosis, there may be no significant discomfort in daily life, so most people do not visit the rehabilitation medicine clinic right away. In reality, the active consideration for rehabilitation medicine treatment begins when walking difficulties arise. When gait becomes problematic, people start to think about professional treatment to correct it. As discussed in previous chapters, starting exercise as early as possible is beneficial. Of course, this exercise does not have to be done exclusively in a rehabilitation medicine clinic. Exercise should begin in any form, but when gait abnormalities start, it is advisable to visit a rehabilitation medicine clinic to discuss specialized rehabilitation therapy.

12. WHAT DOES GOOD REHABILITATION THERAPY LOOK LIKE?

Rehabilitation therapy has specific goals. As explained in previous chapters, it aims to optimize a patient's activities, participation, and quality of life by considering individual functional and environmental factors. The goal is to understand the patient's physical condition and environmental factors, maximize their abilities, and help them manage daily life. So, what does rehabilitation therapy that meets these goals look like?

First, it is personalized for the patient.
Second, it requires a multifaceted analysis.
Third, it involves setting and resetting goals repeatedly.

Personalized Rehabilitation Therapy

Patients with Parkinson's disease undergo "neurodevelopmental rehabilitation therapy." Since their physical problems originate in the brain, this therapy is more complex than simple rehabilitation. The brain, as the control center of our body, affects various areas both mentally and physically when it has issues. The greatest advantage of rehabilitation therapy is that it can be tailored to treat the diverse symptoms of each patient. A therapist is assigned to each patient for one-on-one sessions, observing their condition closely and starting with treatments tailored to them. It's like having a personalized tutor for your body.

Although the diagnosis of Parkinson's disease is the same, the symptoms can vary widely from patient to patient. For example, one patient might struggle with speaking, with their voice becoming muffled and soft. During conversations, others frequently ask them to repeat themselves. This patient would primarily receive voice and speech therapy.

Others might find walking particularly difficult. While they seem to have sufficient strength in their arms and legs, they occasionally lose their balance. For those who work on a computer, fine motor skills in their hands might be an issue, with hand tremors being especially stressful. Thus, the symptoms of Parkinson's disease vary greatly, and rehabilitation must meet each patient's unique needs. The therapy follows general principles but can be applied diversely based on individual conditions, much like getting a custom-tailored suit.

Multifaceted Analysis and Multidisciplinary Treatment

To provide ideal rehabilitation therapy, it is necessary to conduct a comprehensive analysis of the patient.

Case Study: Multidisciplinary Treatment for Dopa Min

Dopa Min, aged 75, was diagnosed with Parkinson's disease 17 years ago. Until five years ago, she managed household chores and socialized with friends. Three years ago, her walking slowed down, and she began to fall frequently. Three months ago, she found it difficult to move at all and struggled with daily activities, prompting a visit to the rehabilitation center. After examining her, several issues were identified. Her difficulty walking was partly due to the progression of Parkinson's disease. However, she also suffered from severe depression. Her lack of motivation made it hard for her to move and perform daily activities. Her appetite decreased, leading to poor nutrition and significant muscle loss.

Dopa Min's treatment plan encompasses all these aspects:
First, since her Parkinson's disease has progressed, appropriate medication is prescribed.
Second, nutritional counseling is conducted. Blood tests identify deficiencies, and a meal plan to increase muscle mass is developed. Supplements are taken if necessary. Proper nutrition is crucial, so support from those around her is essential for balanced dietary intake.
Third, treating depression is vital. Depression can stem from Parkinson's disease itself and makes physical activity and quality of life much harder. For Dopa Min, combining exercise therapy with depression treatment is imperative.

Deterioration in walking ability is one possible result, but there can be multiple underlying causes for this outcome. Rehabilitation therapy isn't just about training for physical activity; it must consider medical, social, and psychological factors. This means looking beyond neurology to include rehabilitation medicine, internal medicine, orthopedics, psychiatry, and other relevant fields. The larger the hospital, the more specialized departments there are. Even within the same department, there are often subspecialties. This allows for deep and detailed treatment of the disease. Additionally, a broad perspective that transcends departmental boundaries is also essential.

Parkinson's disease presents with a variety of complex symptoms. Therefore, analyzing its causes from multiple perspectives and considering various factors for treatment is essential. Rehabilitation for Parkinson's disease requires a team of experts from different fields. This team includes neurologists, rehabilitation physicians, physical therapists, activity therapists, speech therapists, nutritionists, clinical psychologists, nurses, and, importantly, the patient and their family. This is known as a multidisciplinary approach. Each specialist analyzes the patient from their area of expertise, collaborates with other professionals, and sets rehabilitation goals. These goals consider not only the individual's functional aspects but also environmental factors, aiming to find the best treatment for the patient, encompassing both the patient's and their family's needs.

Setting and Reassessing Goals

Two Months into Dopa Min's Treatment.

Dopa Min improved her eating habits, adjusted her medications for depression and Parkinson's, and began serious physical therapy. She recovered faster than the medical team expected. She was enthusiastic about rehabilitation therapy and even exercised at home, seemingly normalizing her daily life.

Two months later, however, she struggled to continue exercising and was confined to bed once more. The culprit was degenerative arthritis in her knee. As her appetite increased, so did her weight, and her intense exercise regime strained her knee. Her knee became swollen, and her pain worsened, leading to increased depression. She no longer wanted to walk.

Parkinson's disease doesn't end with diagnosis and initial treatment. It's a lifelong journey. What is true a month ago might not be true today. Rehabilitation goals must adapt accordingly. Depending on the stage of Parkinson's and the emerging challenges, the goals and content of rehabilitation therapy need to be adjusted. Significant changes in the patient's condition necessitate a thorough reassessment and goal-setting. Even without major changes, patients should be evaluated in detail every three to six months.

Dopa Min's rehabilitation plan changed. Although her ability to walk was similar to two months ago, the cause and specifics had changed. First, her knee needed treatment. X-rays were taken, and she received injections and medication to reduce inflammation and swelling. Her exercise plan was revised to include low-impact activities that put less strain on her knees, along with exercises to strengthen her leg muscles.

Parkinson's rehabilitation is patient and family-centered. It starts with evaluating the patient's Parkinson's symptoms and motor functions. It also involves understanding other medical conditions, social environment, and the role of the family. Effective rehabilitation requires a personalized, multidisciplinary approach with experts from various fields and ongoing goal adjustments.

13. THE CHALLENGES OF REHABILITATION THERAPY

"Doctor, don't talk about unrealistic things. Do you know how hard it is to find a rehab center for someone with Parkinson's?"

Even in the United States and other advanced countries, finding adequate rehabilitation therapy for Parkinson's disease patients can be a significant challenge. Despite having some of the best medical facilities in the world, many Parkinson's patients still struggle to access the rehabilitation therapy they need. As a doctor who emphasizes the importance of exercise for Parkinson's patients, I am acutely aware of the difficulties our patients face in accessing rehabilitation therapy. It pains me to know this. I've pondered over and over why it is so hard to get rehabilitation exercise therapy.

Parkinson's disease is a progressive condition.

Neurological diseases require rehabilitation therapy. For instance, a stroke can cause paralysis of one arm and leg and speech difficulties. Rehabilitation is crucial after acute stroke treatment. Similarly, if there is spinal cord damage leading to lower body paralysis, rehabilitation therapy is essential for returning to daily life.

These conditions are most severe at onset. For example, stroke, which was previously called apoplexy, occurs suddenly, with the initial state being the most critical. Intensive neurological treatment is provided for about a week, followed by rehabilitation therapy. While there may be lingering aftereffects, rehabilitation helps recover muscle strength, cognition, and speech. Inpatient treatment is followed by outpatient rehabilitation, gradually leading to improvement and eventual cessation of therapy.

The national standards for rehabilitation treatment are based on the "date of onset" of the condition. Generally, for brain and nerve disorders, intensive rehabilitation therapy is guaranteed for up to six months from the onset date. In certain cases, hospitalized patients can receive central nervous system developmental rehabilitation therapy twice a day for up to two years. After two to five years, the available rehabilitation treatments become limited. This limitation is based on the belief that the effectiveness of rehabilitation diminishes as more time passes since the onset of the disease. This approach is correct for conditions like stroke or spinal cord injuries.

However, Parkinson's disease is a bit different. When first diagnosed, patients are usually in their best condition. As time goes on, various motor symptoms start to manifest more prominently. Although some patients might experience gait disturbances from the beginning, most initially face only minor inconveniences. By the time our patients truly need rehabilitation therapy, a significant amount of time has often passed since the onset, making it difficult to receive intensive rehabilitation like stroke patients do.

"So, why not start intensive rehabilitation right after diagnosis?"

Early-stage Parkinson's patients often experience little to no difficulty in daily life. Even with a diagnosis, they can usually continue their social and daily activities. Therefore, they rarely visit rehabilitation medicine departments, and when they do, the symptoms are so mild that setting treatment goals is challenging. They might even hear, "Let's start therapy when it gets a bit more severe."

Another challenge is finding specialized Parkinson's rehabilitation centers.

"Where can I get rehabilitation treatment?" Patients often ask this question, but it's not easy to provide a straightforward answer. While many hospitals offer neurological rehabilitation, they mainly cater to inpatients. Outpatient treatment involves long wait times, which can be discouraging for many patients. As a result, many patients end up relying on medication from their neurologists and exploring alternative treatments outside the formal medical system.

If you've ever searched the internet for terms like "Parkinson's disease," "Parkinson's treatment," or "Parkinson's exercise," you've probably come across numerous alternative medicine sites advertised. This doesn't mean all these treatments are ineffective, but some are exaggeratedly advertised and can mislead patients. It's important not to fall prey to marketing tactics that exploit the desperate mindset of Parkinson's patients.

We need to improve the system and establish specialized Parkinson's exercise centers.

Korea boasts an excellent healthcare system, including outstanding rehabilitation therapies. However, Parkinson's disease has unique characteristics that require tailored approaches. Parkinson's rehabilitation should adopt a multidisciplinary approach, considering the individual characteristics of each patient. It would be ideal to have centers that understand the nature of Parkinson's and can provide personalized rehabilitation exercises at every stage of the disease. This should be an integral part of the formal healthcare system. It is also a dream shared by many neurologists.

One day, the system will improve, and specialized Parkinson's exercise centers may pop up in every neighborhood. However, these changes require significant time and financial investment. We can't afford to wait passively. Fortunately, exercise is something that can be done anywhere. Even without a perfect system or fancy centers, you can still exercise effectively. Detailed guidance on how to exercise can be immensely helpful.

14. NEVERTHELESS, KEEP EXERCISING!

We've discussed the goals and ideal approaches for rehabilitation therapy in Parkinson's disease. This chapter might have felt a bit frustrating because it can seem disconnected from reality. Receiving rehabilitation therapy isn't always easy. It would be great if specialists in every field

could focus exclusively on you, observing you meticulously as if under a microscope. However, the reality is that appointments often end as quickly as they begin. When you try to explain your issues, you might hear, "Oh, really? Then you should see a gastroenterologist." They often suggest discussing specific problems with the relevant department.

If I can't get the perfect rehabilitation exercise therapy at the hospital, what should I do?

When the COVID-19 virus spread worldwide, many children couldn't attend school. For a high school senior preparing for college exams, what should they do when schools are closed? Some kids might think, 'Great, time to have fun at home,' while others might decide to study diligently at home despite not being able to go to school. Which student is wiser?

The primary goal of receiving rehabilitation therapy at the hospital is to help you live better in your daily life outside the hospital. Time in the hospital is limited. Even if you receive excellent rehabilitation therapy there, you must continue exercising at home. Just like you practice at home what you learn at school, you need to exercise at home to make it your own. In some ways, students who study hard on their own at home can often learn more deeply and gain greater knowledge.

Exercise should become a part of your daily life. It should be your routine. Start exercising in the comfort of your familiar space. If you keep up with the exercises that suit you, can there be a better time spent? You might feel disappointed if you can't get proper coaching at the hospital. But don't give up. By reading this book carefully and assessing yourself, you can develop your own exercise program. It would be even better with the help of your caregivers. Study together and start exercising. Instead of despairing over real-life challenges, choose what you can do right now.

That's why I began writing this book. If you can pick up jewels just by bending down, there's no need to hesitate because you don't have a grabber.

"So, let's study Parkinson's disease together and make a plan for exercising."

"Don't give up and stay with me until the end!"

PART 4.
DESIGNING THE RIGHT EXERCISE FOR ME

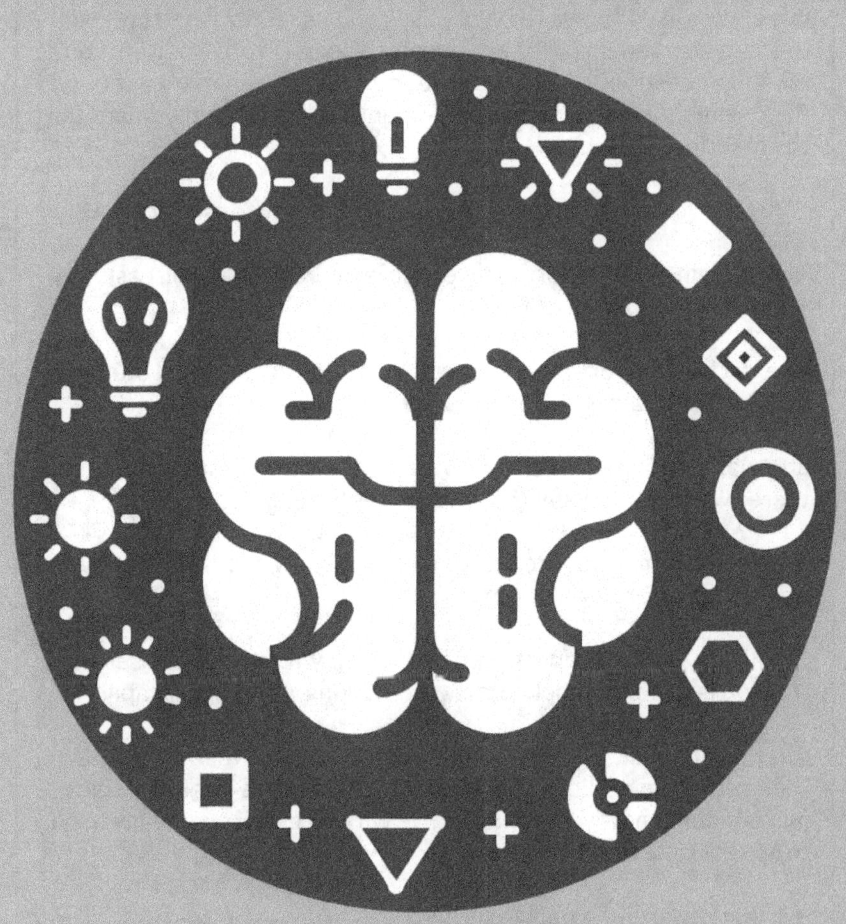

1. MR. PARKINSON, LET'S WALK TOGETHER

James Park Starts Exercising.

I've always liked things to be precise and logical. So, when I asked if exercise was beneficial for Parkinson's disease, Professor Kim didn't take my question lightly. He gave me several research papers on Parkinson's disease and exercise. Thanks to him, I studied hard for the first time in a while.

"Why are you studying so hard these days?" my wife asked curiously.

"I'm studying how important exercise is for Parkinson's disease." Then my wife burst out laughing.

"If exercise is important, you should be exercising, not just studying about it!" she said.

She was right. The conclusion was that exercise is important, yet there I was, sitting down the whole time. I laughed too.

"Professor Kim, I want to start exercising. How should I begin with exercises that are right for me?"

"That's an excellent question. The best way to start exercises that suit you is to begin simply. Start with walking. Just begin simply."

Alright, let's walk. Let's walk. If that's how to start, then let's do it. Parkinson. They called it Parkinson's disease. This strange Englishman's name is now something I'll live with forever. I extend my hand to Mr. Parkinson.

"Mr. Parkinson, let's walk together."

Starting Exercise

The previous chapter may have been boring and difficult. It's okay to skim through it. In short, exercise is very important in Parkinson's disease. You can read the entire book and carefully plan your exercise routine before starting, but I emphasize that the most important thing is to 'just start.' First, get up and begin exercising. Then, adjust your routine using the book as a reference to find the exercises that suit you best. So, how should you start exercising?

Benefits of Walking Outside

The first benefit is sunlight. Sunlight is a blessing. For modern people who mostly stay indoors, sunlight is like a tonic. It is associated with vitamin D and helps strengthen our bones. It also boosts our immune system. Especially when you get sunlight early in the morning, it can help you sleep better at night. This is called light therapy. Exposure to bright sunlight can also prevent depression. Imagine a world filled with sunlight. Doesn't just thinking about it make you feel better? Sunlight is a jewel-like gift from God to humanity.

The second benefit is connection. Going outside allows you to connect with nature. You can physically feel the changes of the four seasons. In spring, the gentle breeze blows, and fresh green sprouts emerge. The ground that was frozen all winter becomes soft. In summer, you might sweat profusely after just a short walk, and then you can take a break in the shade of a tree. The breeze cools the sweat on your forehead. Birds sing. Autumn, the queen of seasons, is even better. The world transforms into a vibrant display. The high autumn sky is beautiful. Winter also has its charm. The cold winter wind feels like it cuts through your skin, and the dried-up branches seem to grow stronger in the cold. There are people and pets on the streets. Hearing children laugh and seeing people of all sorts pass by makes you feel alive. Your presence in this society is valuable. By going outside, you can connect with both nature and the community.

The third benefit is comprehensive training for daily life skills. Walking outside stimulates your vision, hearing, and touch, which improves brain function. These stimuli, combined with emotions, also help enhance memory. Various stimuli improve physical responsiveness. As you walk, you might encounter puddles or have to avoid rocks. When you see an approaching bicycle, you step aside. Walking on a hard path is different from walking on a muddy one. You learn how your body should react when walking on wide or narrow paths. When it rains, you walk with an umbrella. When the rain stops, you fold the umbrella. When you're tired, you find a bench to sit on. Sitting, standing, putting your shoes back on, and walking—all these are daily life skills. Exercise and rehabilitation aim to improve these skills. Walking outside naturally trains these skills.

I have great respect for a senior doctor couple who left their comfortable and stable lives in Korea to volunteer in a country with different medical challenges. Their dedication and service to that country were heartfelt. Once, when they visited Korea after a long time, we arranged to meet. They walked five subway stations to our meeting place.

"Why? Was it difficult to take the subway?"

"Dr. Kim, we were reminded of how unique and special our surroundings are."

"The trees along the street, the pavement, the people passing by. Walking on such safe and lovely streets made us so happy that we held hands and walked."

Their response was truly moving. Sometimes, we are so close to something valuable that we fail to see it. The paths that seem so familiar and insignificant to us are filled with someone's dedication and effort. Small sculptures, neatly trimmed trees, benches placed at potentially difficult spots, and flowers visible from those benches. Let's walk a bit more and enjoy this beautiful world with gratitude.

2. EFFECTIVE WALKING METHODS FOR PARKINSON'S DISEASE

Remember these three effective walking methods for Parkinson's:

1. Walk until you're out of breath.
2. Walk with long strides.
3. Swing your arms vigorously while walking.

The more you walk, the better. If you're going to walk, it might as well be effective. What are the effective walking methods for Parkinson's?

First, walk until you're out of breath.

Many studies have shown positive effects from brisk walking. Referring to the WHO's recommendation from the previous chapter, engage in "moderate-intensity" aerobic exercise. Moderate intensity means walking briskly at about 3 to 4 miles per hour. Brisk walking is great, but Parkinson's patients should not rush. Trying to walk fast can cause your posture to become unsteady and increase forward lean. Rapid steps are also a symptom of Parkinson's.

Walking fast is a very good exercise, but think of it as walking until you're out of breath rather than walking quickly. Medically, walking until you're out of breath means using 50-80% of your heart rate reserve. When we exercise, our heart starts to beat faster. The difference between your maximum heart rate and your resting heart rate is your heart rate reserve. Simply put, if resting is a 1 and maximum exertion is a 5, aim to walk at a 3-4 level of intensity. If you're not out of breath and your heart isn't beating faster, the exercise is less effective.

Second, walk with long strides.

One characteristic of Parkinson's walking is that steps get shorter the more you walk, resulting in shuffling steps. Practice intentionally taking longer strides. You can start by walking with long, slow strides at the beginning and then gradually return to your natural pace. During the last 10 minutes of your walk, practice long strides again. Gradually increase the time you spend walking with long strides.

Short strides are typical in Parkinson's. If you find your steps getting shorter, pause for a moment. Imagine drawing a line on the ground in front of you. Practice stepping over the line at 2-foot intervals. If there are actual marks or lines on the ground, use them. Walking with long strides also stimulates the brain more. This technique is also helpful for overcoming gait difficulties later on by using visual cues.

Third, swing your arms vigorously while walking.

In typical Parkinson's, the disease often starts on one side of the body. Tremors, slowness, and stiffness are usually more pronounced on one side. Naturally, we don't think about swinging our arms while walking. It's not something the brain consciously controls. In Parkinson's, the arm swing on the affected side is reduced. So, make a conscious effort to swing your arms vigorously while walking, especially the affected side.

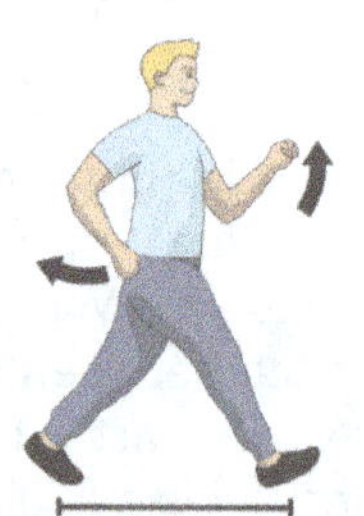

Walk briskly with long strides, swinging your arms vigorously.

To summarize, walk with long strides, swinging both arms vigorously, and walk until you're out of breath. This is not about walking unconsciously but intentionally using your brain. Thinking and walking stimulates the brain more. Walking also helps balance your body, strengthens your core muscles, and improves posture. It enhances lower body strength, which helps prevent orthostatic hypotension. Most importantly, walking activates cognitive areas, helping prevent dementia. Walking vigorously also leads to better sleep and reduces depression. I hope you experience the happiness that comes from walking.

How long should you walk? The answer varies greatly from person to person. Since everyone's fitness level is different, there is no one-size-fits-all answer. Especially when starting, it's good to begin gently. Walk for 30 minutes out and 30 minutes back. It's okay to walk slowly. Spend an hour outside walking. Gradually increase the intensity and duration over time. Once you're comfortable with walking, try walking "vigorously, with long strides, and swinging your arms." It may be challenging to walk like this for an entire hour. Set a goal to walk like this from a park bench to a streetlight and gradually expand the distance you walk consciously and attentively.

Walking for an hour may be difficult. Even walking itself might be challenging. That's okay. When you're tired, sit on a bench and rest. Sitting on a bench, feel the sunlight, watch passing cars, and listen to children playing. Feel the breeze and the changing seasons. This itself is excellent exercise.

"How about it? Is it doable? Don't overthink how to exercise with Parkinson's."
"Set a time each day, like going to work, and walk outside for an hour."
"Just start. It will make your life vibrant and filled with interaction with the world."

3. DESIGNING THE RIGHT EXERCISE FOR ME: UNDERSTANDING MYSELF AND MY DISEASE

"I've started walking for exercise. I walk for an hour every day, sometimes even two. Getting out of the house has brought new energy into my life."

"When I stayed home, negative thoughts kept creeping in, and I started feeling more and more withdrawn. I worried that people would judge my gait. I felt embarrassed by my trembling hands while walking."

"But those feelings were fleeting. More often, people give me encouraging looks, telling me to keep up the good work. Honestly, most people don't care how I look. I felt isolated at home, but stepping outside, I feel truly alive."

"Walking is great, but I want to exercise more systematically. How can I do that?"

Designing the Right Exercise for Me

For those of you who have started walking regularly, you're doing a great job. However, you might want to exercise more systematically. In this chapter, we will learn how to design the most suitable exercise for yourself.

The first step in doing this is to 'know yourself and know your disease.'

We think we know ourselves well. And that's true; no one knows us better than we do. However, our knowledge about ourselves is highly subjective. To exercise effectively, you need to know yourself 'objectively.'

Then, you need to understand yourself subjectively. What does it mean to know yourself objectively? Let's answer the following questions one by one. Don't just think about them; write them down. Writing helps organize our thoughts.

"Nosce te ipsum (Know thyself, Socrates)."

Creating Your Own Disease Analysis Chart

Write down the history of your Parkinson's disease. It might seem daunting, but answering these questions will help you understand your disease better. When were you diagnosed with Parkinson's disease? What symptoms did you have when you first went to the hospital? What symptoms do you have now?

Also, write down any other diseases you have besides Parkinson's. Do you have chronic diseases like diabetes, hypertension, hyperlipidemia, or heart disease? List the medications for each disease, distinguishing between Parkinson's medications and others.

Now think about your personal and social roles. What is your occupation? What tasks do you currently need to do? Write down any symptoms you want to improve. Also, think about what you want to do. Whether it's small daily tasks or big planned activities, write them down.

When exercising, you might feel disappointed seeing yourself less capable than before and noticing worsening symptoms. You may feel discouraged, embarrassed about what others might think, and find it hard to keep going. However, exercise is not a hobby when you have Parkinson's disease. It is essential treatment to improve the disease and achieve better outcomes. Stay determined and start exercising with a strong will. Write down your disease and symptoms. Refer to Daisy's chart and create your own disease analysis chart.

Disease Analysis Chart

Diagnosis Date	
Initial Symptoms	
Current Symptoms	
Other Diseases	
Parkinson's Medications	
Other Medications	
Occupation	
Necessary Tasks	
Desired Activities	
Symptoms to Improve	

April 7, 2023 Daisy's Disease Analysis Chart	
Diagnosis Date	March 2016
Initial Symptoms	Tremor in left hand
Current Symptoms	Tremor, slower hand movements, short and fast steps, hunched back
Other Diseases	Hypertension, diabetes, hyperlipidemia, degenerative knee joint disease
Parkinson's Medications	Sinemet 100/25mg three times a day, Requip 2mg three times a day
Other Medications	Morning: medications for hypertension, diabetes, and hyperlipidemia; Night: sleeping pills; Occasionally: medication for joint disease
Occupation	Homemaker
Necessary Tasks	Household chores, preparing meals for husband and son, occasionally looking after grandchild
Desired Activities	Cooking, painting, traveling
Symptoms to Improve	Gait issues, insomnia, depression

4. EXERCISE GOALS AND PRECAUTIONS BY STAGE OF PROGRESSION

Parkinson's disease progresses slowly. It is categorized into five stages using the Hoehn and Yahr scale. You need to roughly determine your stage to evaluate your progression. This might be an unpleasant task, but it helps you find and enjoy what you can do. Understanding your vulnerabilities allows you to focus on training those areas.

Hoehn and Yahr Stages of Parkinson's Disease Progression

Stage 1: Symptoms like slowness or tremors are present on only one side of the body.
Stage 2: Symptoms affect both sides of the body.
Stage 3: Changes in walking and balance begin to occur.
Stage 4: The disease has progressed further, and assistance with daily activities is needed.
Stage 5: Significant help from others is required, and independent movement becomes very difficult.

"When should I start exercising?"
"Stage 1? Stage 2?"

The answer is 10 years before diagnosis. The brain's degeneration begins about 10 years before Parkinson's symptoms appear. By the time symptoms manifest, many dopamine cells are already lost. Therefore, starting exercise therapy at Stage 1, even if symptoms are mild, is advisable.

Hoehn and Yahr Stages	Symptoms	Exercise Goals	Precautions
1	Symptoms are present on one side only	1. Prevent decreased activity levels 2. Improve physical capabilities	1. Enjoy your favorite exercises 2. No special exercise restrictions 3. Avoid injuries from strenuous activities 4. Focus on correct posture
2	Symptoms are present on both sides. Posture is stooped		
3	Shuffling steps. Occasionally almost falls Speech is slurred and voice becomes softer. Often chokes on food or liquids	1. Prevent falls 2. Maintain independence in daily activities	1. The most important thing is to avoid falling 2. Include respiratory muscle training: engage in activities like singing or reciting poetry
4	Frequently falls Uses a wheelchair in crowded places Speech is difficult to understand Frequently chokes	1. Enhance daily living skills 2. Prevent pneumonia 3. Prevent contractures 4. Prevent bedsores	1. Always have a caregiver accompany you during exercise 2. Train for independent daily living
5	Always uses a wheelchair Mostly bedridden		1. Minimize time spent lying down 2. Joint stretching to prevent contractures

Exercise Goals for Stages 1 and 2

1. Prevent decline in activity.
2. Improve physical capacity.

Most patients are diagnosed at Stages 1 or 2. After diagnosis and starting levodopa medication, the body's condition improves significantly. Parkinson's disease is progressive. Gradually, motor skills become dull and uncomfortable. Hence, in the early stages, preventing a decline in activity is the first exercise goal. Habitualize active movement and exercise as much as possible.

In the early stages, make extra efforts to stay active in your daily life. Move more on purpose, try tasks you didn't do before, and do your usual activities more enthusiastically. The shock of diagnosis and psychological withdrawal can make it hard to stay active. Change your mindset a bit and make an effort to move.

Right now is a precious time in your life to move actively. Attend gatherings, visit nearby cafes with a good atmosphere, and travel with close friends. If you have hobbies you enjoy, immerse yourself in them. Don't reduce your range of activities; instead, expand them with enjoyable things. Don't hesitate to learn and face new challenges.

Second, improving physical abilities has multiple meanings. On a smaller scale, it means strengthening muscles and increasing joint flexibility. On a broader scale, it means enabling our bodies to perform more tasks and actions. Throughout the day, we move a lot and engage in various activities.

Seven-year-olds dart around effortlessly and do quick somersaults. Twenty-year-olds can climb ladders to fix roofs and lift heavy bags of groceries. They swim in streams and surf at the beach. On snowy days, they carefully shovel snow to avoid slipping. All these movements and actions depend on physical abilities, which determine whether we can perform them or not.

As we age, our movements and activities become simpler. Additionally, the strength and function of our musculoskeletal system are not what they used to be. If you have Parkinson's disease, your motor functions may decline even further. While strength and flexibility may decrease, it's important to make an effort to move your joints to their fullest extent. Increasing physical capabilities through various movements and tasks in daily life is crucial in the early stages of Parkinson's.

In stages 1 and 2 of Parkinson's, exercise abilities are similar to those of adults without the disease. If you have a favorite sport, enjoy it to the fullest. There are no specific exercises you need to avoid. However, if a particular exercise causes joint pain, it's best to steer clear of it. While there are no exercises you can't do, engaging in overly strenuous activities that could injure your body is not advisable. Fractures or ligament injuries require recovery time and minimized movement, which can lead to a rapid decline in physical abilities. Therefore, it's important to exercise safely.

Exercise Recommendations for Stages 1 and 2

The foundation of exercise should be aerobic activities, supplemented by strength training, especially for core muscles. Aerobic exercise is highly recommended because it trains your heart and lungs. Improved cardiovascular endurance helps prevent tachycardia syndrome and pneumonia. It enhances overall fitness and blood circulation throughout the body, and it's excellent for alleviating depression and sleep disorders. Choose activities you enjoy, such as walking, running, cycling, swimming, or hiking. The more you enjoy it, the more likely you are to do it regularly. Try to see exercise as a fun activity rather than a burden.

If symptoms are asymmetrical, engage in balanced exercises to prevent muscle atrophy on the affected side. Well-trained core muscles in the early stages are essential to compensate for future balance issues. Since stooped posture is common in the early stages, practice standing straight and stretching your back muscles to prevent them from atrophying.

Parkinson's can affect the autonomic nervous system, leading to dizziness or a drop in blood pressure when standing up. Increase lower body muscle mass through strength training, which is excellent for preventing orthostatic hypotension. Exercises like squats, stair climbing, and hiking are great for strengthening the lower body. Using a rowing machine, which mimics the action of rowing a boat, is particularly suitable for lower body strength. If you experience dizziness while standing, a rowing machine is highly recommended.

Exercise Goals in Stage 3

1. Preventing falls.
2. Maintaining independence in daily life.

In stage 3, the primary goals are to prevent falls and maintain independence in daily life. The most important objective is to avoid falling. Even if you walk well most of the time, a sudden fall can happen. Falling and sustaining a severe injury is the biggest threat to someone with Parkinson's. This issue is not exclusive to Parkinson's; it's a major concern for the elderly in general. Many traumatic brain injuries are linked to falls. Even without severe trauma, repeated head impacts can lead to chronic subdural hematoma. If an elderly person suddenly has trouble walking and experiences incontinence, brain hemorrhage should be considered.

Falls can cause not only brain injuries but also fractures and joint problems. Recovery is slower as we age. Prolonged periods of immobility can lead to severe joint contractures and degeneration. Therefore, avoiding falls and injuries in daily life is of utmost importance. As Parkinson's progresses, walking difficulties become more frequent. Engage in exercises that help prevent falls.

The second goal is to maintain independence in daily life. As you become more passive and your motor skills decrease, you may find yourself relying more on others for daily tasks. This is natural, but you should strive to do as much as possible on your own. It's also necessary to modify your living environment to make it easier to live independently.

Exercise Recommendations for Stage 3

Walking is the basic form of aerobic exercise, but if safety can be ensured, walking in a swimming pool is excellent. For those with severe walking difficulties, indoor cycling is a good option. As the back tends to hunch and vision narrows, diligently stretch your back, neck, and shoulders. Engage in resistance training to maintain lower body strength. Training posture and balance should be key goals, and always prioritize safety to avoid falls while exercising.

Ms. Daisy Wildflower's Story in Hoehn and Yahr Stage 3

Ms. Wildflower loves cooking. Her greatest joy is preparing meals and serving them to others. However, after developing Parkinson's, cooking became a challenge. Reaching for dishes on high shelves and opening small spice jars were frustrating tasks due to her hand difficulties.

With wisdom and cooperation, her family made adjustments. They placed dishes within her reach and replaced the gas stove with an electric one to reduce the risk. Knowing it would be hard for her to stand for long periods, they put a small table in the kitchen where she could sit while chopping vegetables and mixing salads. Hard-to-open spice jars were replaced with larger ones, and lighter pots and pans were purchased. The kitchen was simplified, and all clutter that could trip her was removed. Ms. Wildflower found cooking much easier and was thrilled to be able to cook again, even if the meals weren't as elaborate as before. She was happy to discover she could still enjoy cooking.

Patients in Stage 3 of Parkinson's disease should exercise with a focus on preventing falls. It is essential to engage in physical activities that help avoid falls while also strengthening areas of weakness to maintain independence in daily life. Additionally, it's important to make changes to your surroundings to ensure a safe environment.

Exercise Goals in Stages 4 and 5

1. Training for daily living skills.
2. Preventing various diseases.

In stages 4 and 5, the exercise goals are to train for daily living skills and prevent other diseases. The focus is on maximizing the ability to perform necessary movements in daily life despite limited exercise capacity.

In stages 4 and 5, aside from Parkinson's, pneumonia, contractures, and pressure sores can also significantly impact both quality of life and life expectancy. Therefore, efforts to prevent these conditions are essential.

Exercise Recommendations for Stage 4

In stage 4, it is crucial to avoid falls even more carefully. Always have a caregiver present during exercise. In this stage, adding diligent joint stretching is very important. When joint movement is restricted, the range of motion decreases. If you don't use it, you lose it. Stretch all joints to their fullest extent, practicing standing straight regularly. Since dizziness is common when standing, always have a caregiver nearby. As Parkinson's progresses, maintaining muscle strength through resistance training is necessary. Performing daily tasks requires coordinated muscle use and smooth movements. Parkinson's can disrupt this coordination, making movement more difficult without muscle strength. Therefore, aim to maintain muscle mass through resistance training.

Hoehn and Yahr Stage 4 Exercise Story: Dopa Min

Dopa Min often wakes up at dawn needing to use the bathroom. This routine is a struggle every time. Getting out of her high bed is difficult, fumbling for the light switch, and making her way to the bathroom is a challenge. She often feels dizzy and has stumbled several times on the way there. She frequently wakes her husband to help her . During the day however, it's not as hard for her to get to the bathroom.

Dopa Min set specific goals to be able to go to the bathroom by herself at night. She focused on lower body strength exercises and practiced sitting and standing movements at home. These exercises helped her stabilize her balance, making her trips to the bathroom much steadier. Additionally, she replaced her high bed with a lower one, allowing her feet to touch the floor when sitting, making it easier to stand up. She placed a small lamp within reach so she could turn on the light immediately and avoid darkness. She ensured the path to the bathroom was clear of obstacles and left a dim light on

---

> for safety. Now, Dopa Min isn't afraid to go to the bathroom at night without her husband.

Stage 5 Exercise Suggestions

At Stage 5, caregiver assistance is crucial. The most important thing is to minimize the time spent lying down. Make an effort to sit up and regularly spend time standing with support. Staying in bed too long can increase dizziness and the risk of aspiration pneumonia due to choking. There is also the risk of pressure sores on the hips or ankles from prolonged lying.

Joint exercises need assistance. It's beneficial to move each joint at least once a day. If you notice any joint becoming stiff, pay extra attention to exercising that joint.

Singing at any stage is highly beneficial. Singing loudly helps with breathing exercises, pronunciation training, and prevents choking. If you are not confident in singing, try reciting poetry. Select good poems and read them slowly and loudly. This can be reminiscent of poetry readings or open mic nights where participants read poems aloud to an audience. Standing tall and projecting your voice as if you're on stage can help relieve stress and enrich your cultural knowledge.

5. THE PRACTICE OF EXERCISE: PREPARATION - MAIN EXERCISE - FINISHING

The exercise routine is broadly divided into three stages: Preparation, Main Exercise, and Conclusion.

Preparation

1. Prioritize exercise
2. Set a time: Start about an hour after eating and taking medication, such as 9 AM, 2 PM, or 7 PM
3. Wear comfortable clothes and sneakers

Main Exercise: Four Parts

1. Aerobic Exercise
2. Resistance Exercise
3. Posture and Balance Exercise
4. Respiratory Muscle Exercise

Finishing

1. Rest well as part of the exercise process
2. Keep a journal of grateful moments
3. Practice meditation and breathing techniques

1. Preparation Process

The first step in preparation is to make exercise a priority. Consider it a vital part of your treatment. If you've decided to exercise after reading this book, you've made an excellent decision! You've taken the first step towards exercise therapy.

Make exercise a priority and schedule it. While daily exercise is best, aim to exercise at least three times a week. Choose a time when you can focus without interruptions. It's best for Parkinson's patients to exercise when their medication levels are stable.

Start exercising at least 20 minutes after breakfast and medication. For instance, if you eat breakfast around 8 AM, starting exercise at 9 AM is ideal. Exercising after eating and taking your medication is important. While exercising on an empty stomach can have benefits such as reducing body fat, it is not suitable for Parkinson's patients. Exercising on an empty stomach can cause your blood sugar levels to drop quickly, increasing the risk of dizziness. Additionally, prolonged exercise on an empty stomach can lead to muscle loss as your body might start using protein for energy. Therefore, it is essential for Parkinson's patients to have a meal before exercising.

Begin exercising at least 20 minutes after taking Parkinson's medication, like levodopa. If you don't feel the medication's effect, wait a bit longer and exercise when the medication is working well. Exercising when levodopa is effective reduces muscle tension and increases flexibility, minimizing the risk of falls and injuries.

Thus, when planning your exercise, prioritize regular meal and medication times. A balanced diet is essential for effective exercise. Don't just have a quick meal; include plenty of vegetables, alternating fish and meat, and enjoy various greens. Chewing well and savoring your food is the first step of your exercise routine.

Wear comfortable clothes for exercise. Always wear socks. Choose lightweight, non-slip sneakers. Keep your hands free. Carry your phone and water bottle in a side bag. If you need a cane, don't forget to bring it.

During exercise time, focus solely on exercising. Don't try to multitask. Don't exercise while watching a video on your phone or checking text messages. This isn't just for Parkinson's patients but for everyone. Many accidents happen due to inattention. Parkinson's patients should be extra cautious. Remember, focus on one thing at a time.

You should focus on exercising only when it's time to exercise. Don't try to multitask, like leaving eggs on the stove while you work out. You'll end up burning the eggs and not exercising properly. Try not to answer phone calls during your workout. Most calls can wait until you're done. If you absolutely must take a call, stop exercising and sit down properly to answer it. Especially avoid watching videos on your phone or checking messages while walking. This advice isn't just for Parkinson's patients, but for everyone, as many accidents occur due to distractions. Parkinson's patients should be especially careful. Remember, do one thing at a time.

Parkinson's is a Friend, Not an Enemy.

When diagnosed with Parkinson's and beginning treatment, many people think of the disease as an enemy to be defeated. This isn't the case. Parkinson's is not our enemy. Parkinson's is like a friend who's a bit difficult to deal with. This friend sometimes prevents you from going where you want and feels like a heavy burden on your back. The purpose of exercise isn't to defeat Parkinson's and win a battle. The more you arm yourself and rush into the fight, the more exhausted and depleted you'll feel.

Parkinson's isn't an adversary; it's a friend. We need to acknowledge Parkinson's as a companion and gently coax it along as we go about our lives. This is the mindset you should have for exercise therapy.

2. Starting Your Exercise Routine

As mentioned at the beginning of Chapter 4, simply going outside for a walk is an excellent form of exercise. If you have a favorite sport, sweating it out with enthusiasm is also great. Dancing and singing at a community center can be enjoyable and beneficial forms of exercise. The best exercise is one you can enjoy and do consistently. As mentioned in Chapter 3, any exercise can have great benefits. Be open-minded about different types of exercise.

However, if you want to be more systematic, plan your exercise to include four areas: aerobic exercise, resistance training, balance and posture exercises, and breathing exercises. It's ideal to incorporate exercises from each area every day. If you can't dedicate a lot of time, divide your workouts by day of the week.

(1) Aerobic Exercise

Aerobic exercise involves continuous movement of large muscle groups with sufficient oxygen supply. Examples include walking, running, swimming, biking, and hiking. Start with walking as described earlier. When walking, aim for a "big stride," "swing your arms widely," and "walk briskly." For Parkinson's patients, indoor cycling is also a great aerobic exercise. Even those in the later stages of the disease who experience freezing episodes and find walking difficult can often manage cycling quite well. If you feel you're not getting enough exercise, try indoor cycling. Swimming, hiking, running, and various ball games are also excellent aerobic exercises. Choose the safest and most stable activities based on your physical condition and the progression of Parkinson's.

(2) Resistance Exercise

Resistance exercise, also known as strength training, involves activities designed to improve muscle strength. These exercises are commonly performed at fitness centers using various equipment, but they can also be done with simple tools like resistance bands. Additionally, exercises that use your own body weight, known as body-weight exercises, are a form of resistance training. This type of exercise is highly beneficial for increasing muscle mass and enhancing strength. Importantly, it is excellent for preventing osteoporosis. By engaging the core muscles, resistance exercise helps maintain posture and balance. There are many exercises suitable for patients with limited mobility. These can be performed while sitting or lying down, making them appropriate for Parkinson's patients at all stages of the disease.

It's helpful to have specific guidance when starting resistance exercises. There are many instructional videos online. One highly recommended resource is the booklet "Exercise for Parkinson's Patients" by the Korean Movement Disorder Society. This book, created by experts through extensive research and clinical experience, is a valuable guide.

(3) Posture and Balance Exercises

Posture and balance exercises naturally complement aerobic and resistance training. When walking, maintaining good posture and balance while increasing your stride length is excellent for further improving posture and balance. Additionally, resistance training strengthens muscles, particularly core muscles, which are crucial for maintaining posture and balance. Besides these, specific posture and balance exercises can be beneficial, and for Parkinson's disease, slow-motion exercises like Tai Chi are recommended.

Tai Chi is frequently mentioned as a therapeutic exercise for Parkinson's disease. This ancient Chinese martial art, often seen practiced slowly in parks, might seem unusual, especially if you picture the flashy moves from martial arts movies. However, the goal of Tai Chi is not to engage in combat but to move slowly and shift the body's weight gradually. The movements of the arms and legs might appear independent, but they come together to form a harmonious sequence.

Parkinson's disease is characterized by slowed movements. It might seem logical to focus on quick movements for exercise, so the idea of practicing slow movements like Tai Chi might seem counterintuitive. However, slow movements are actually much more challenging than fast ones. Each movement requires careful, deliberate coordination of the arms and legs, promoting fluidity and balance. It's akin to meditative exercise. Learning Tai Chi well requires about three to six months of practice. Instead of feeling pressured to master numerous movements, it's better to start slowly and appreciate the art of moving gracefully.

Another great exercise for posture and balance is calisthenics. Many older Americans might remember calisthenics from school, a form of exercise involving rhythmic movements and bodyweight exercises, often performed in groups. Calisthenics is beneficial for Parkinson's patients because it's not too fast-paced and involves shifting body weight and using joints, making it ideal for improving posture and balance. Yoga, combined with meditation, is also an excellent exercise. Dancing to slow music can be as enjoyable and effective as Tai Chi for improving posture and balance.

(4) Respiratory Muscle Exercises

One crucial aspect of managing Parkinson's disease is strengthening the respiratory muscles. Proper breathing and clear speech are vital. Parkinson's disease can lead to symptoms like unclear speech, a softer voice, and difficulties swallowing, which might cause coughing or choking. Although termed respiratory muscle exercises, these exercises target the muscles from the mouth to the lungs. At some point, speech might become slurred, speaking speed might increase, and the voice may become quieter, hindering effective communication. Additionally, Parkinson's can cause the vocal cords to tremble, making speech sound stuttered. Choking while swallowing can lead to coughing and the risk of food entering the lungs, potentially causing pneumonia, a severe and often fatal condition for Parkinson's patients.

The best respiratory muscle exercise is singing. Singing engages the vocal cords and controls the muscles that manage breathing, thereby enhancing lung capacity. Singing in an upright posture engages the abdominal muscles and straightens the back. For this exercise, choose songs with varying pitches that aren't too fast—classical songs, hymns, or even slow country songs work well. Don't worry about perfecting the song or keeping the perfect rhythm. Simply enjoy singing and focus on exercising the respiratory and vocal muscles.

Reciting poetry is also recommended. Prepare a poem, write it down, and recite it as if performing at a "poetry night" event. Stand or sit upright, and recite each line loudly and clearly, emphasizing each word. The speed isn't important; focus on controlling your breath and speaking loudly and clearly. Record yourself reciting the poem with your smartphone—it can make for a fun and memorable experience.

3. Finishing Your Workout

After exercising, it's crucial to properly wind down. Don't just stop and drink water—finish with intention. Think of it as a ritual to thoughtfully conclude your session. Write in a journal about today's workout, noting any enjoyable moments or things you're grateful for. If you're not used to writing, that's okay—you don't have to write it down. If you have a religious practice, taking time to pray or meditate can be beneficial. Even just spending 10 minutes with your eyes closed, breathing deeply, and praising yourself for completing your workout can be very rewarding.

When winding down, it's important to focus on positive thoughts. There may have been frustrating moments during your workout—times when things didn't go well and you felt embarrassed or discouraged. But when you're wrapping up your exercise, make sure to give your brain positive signals instead of negative feedback. One of the easiest ways to end on a positive note is to write down three things you're grateful for. It doesn't matter if they're the same as yesterday. If nothing particular comes to mind, jot down something funny or interesting you noticed. Think of three positive things and write them down briefly.

If you want to take your meditation further, I recommend trying "mindfulness meditation." Created by Dr. Jon Kabat-Zinn, mindfulness meditation is about building the muscle of your mind. It allows you to step back and observe your surroundings and reality without being overwhelmed. It's about recognizing and accepting your current thoughts and feelings. Meditation might seem daunting, but it can be done quite easily. There are many methods, so find the one that suits you best. If you're new to this, follow these steps:

Mindfulness meditation starts with breathing and then moves to meditating on your body from an objective perspective. Sit comfortably with your mouth closed and breathe through your nose. Use the 4-4-6 breathing method: breathe in deeply for 4 seconds, hold your breath for 4 seconds, then exhale slowly through your mouth for 6 seconds. Repeat this about five times.

Next, either lying down or sitting comfortably with your eyes closed, imagine stepping out of your body and looking at yourself. Picture yourself in a peaceful place, like lying on a sunny beach. Focus on each part of your body, starting from your toes and moving up to your ankles, calves, knees, thighs, hands, arms, belly, chest, neck, and head. Notice how each part feels. If your arm is trembling, don't think, "Oh no, why is my arm shaking again?" Instead, observe as an outsider: "My right arm is trembling while at rest." If there's pain, think, "My left knee hurts," maintaining a balanced perspective on your body. This process is called a "body scan." After about 10 minutes, conclude your meditation.

Mindfulness meditation is great after exercise, but it's also beneficial to do it every morning when you wake up or at night before you go to sleep. Use your breath to calm your mind and observe your body as an outsider while lying down. Many studies show that mindfulness meditation helps with stress, insomnia, depression, and chronic pain. Since you're already lying down, adding mindfulness meditation to your routine can be highly beneficial for Parkinson's patients.

6. 12 RESISTANCE EXERCISES FOR PARKINSON'S PATIENTS

These resistance exercises are great for Parkinson's patients. You can do them even if you have balance or walking issues, and they're perfect for a quick workout in an office chair or before bed. The exercises include both seated and lying-down routines, all illustrated with pictures by the talented artist Haak, who generously created them to support Parkinson's patients. I'm very grateful for his contribution.

Equipment Needed

A sturdy chair (without wheels, heavy enough not to slide easily)
Comfortable clothing
Well-fitting shoes with non-slip soles

Six Seated Exercises

1. Butterfly Dance
2. Arm Raises with Shoulder Circles
3. Energetic Leg Stretches
4. Heel Alignment
5. Seated Wall Push
6. Side Stretch with Interlaced Fingers

Six Lying Down Exercises

1. Upper Abdominal Crunch
2. Cobra Stretch
3. Scissor Leg Lifts
4. Chest Opener
5. Prone Thigh Lift
6. Stretching Like a Starfish

Six Seated Exercises

1. Butterfly Dance

a. Sit up straight in a chair and stretch both arms out to the sides.
b. Keep your chest open and hold this position for 10 seconds.
c. Slowly lower your arms to about a 30-40 degree angle.
d. Hold for 10 seconds, then raise your arms back to a straight line.
e. Repeat this movement 10 times, maintaining tension in your arms without letting them go limp.
f. You can also hold dumbbells or water bottles in each hand for added resistance.

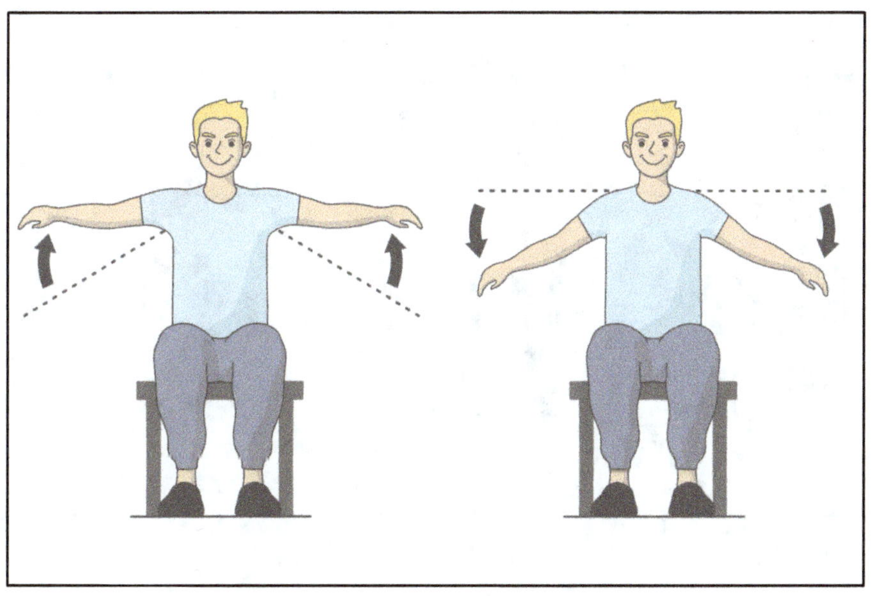

2. Arm Raises with Shoulder Circles

a. Sit with your back straight against the chair back, which should be against a wall.
b. Stretch both arms forward at shoulder height and hold for 10 seconds.
c. Raise your arms upward, keeping them close to your ears, and hold for 10 seconds.
d. Slowly bring your arms down in a wide circle along the wall.
e. Repeat these movements slowly 10 times.

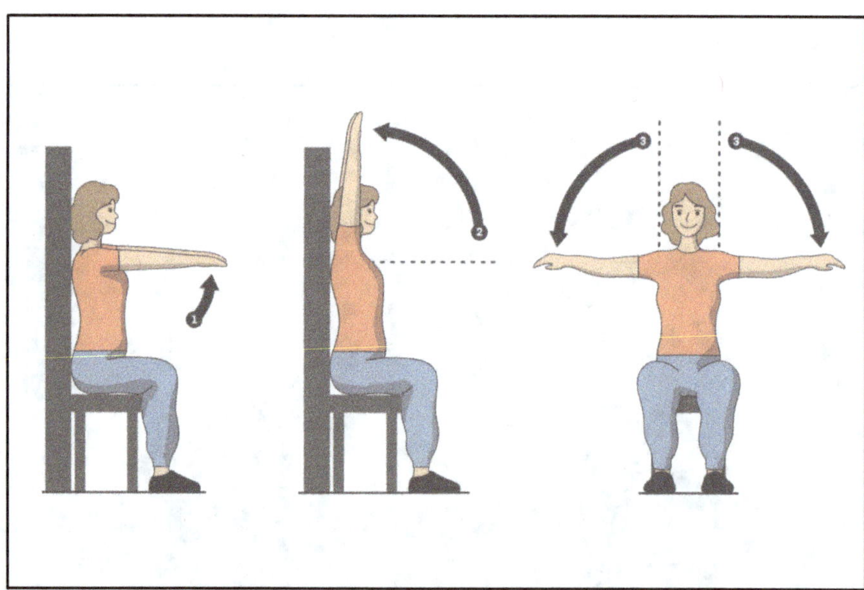

3. Energetic Leg Stretches

a. Sit up straight in a chair.
b. Lift your right thigh, then extend your knee fully forward and hold for 10 seconds.
c. Slowly rotate your right ankle clockwise and counterclockwise.
d. Lower your leg slowly and repeat this movement 5 times.
e. Repeat the same steps with your left leg 5 times.

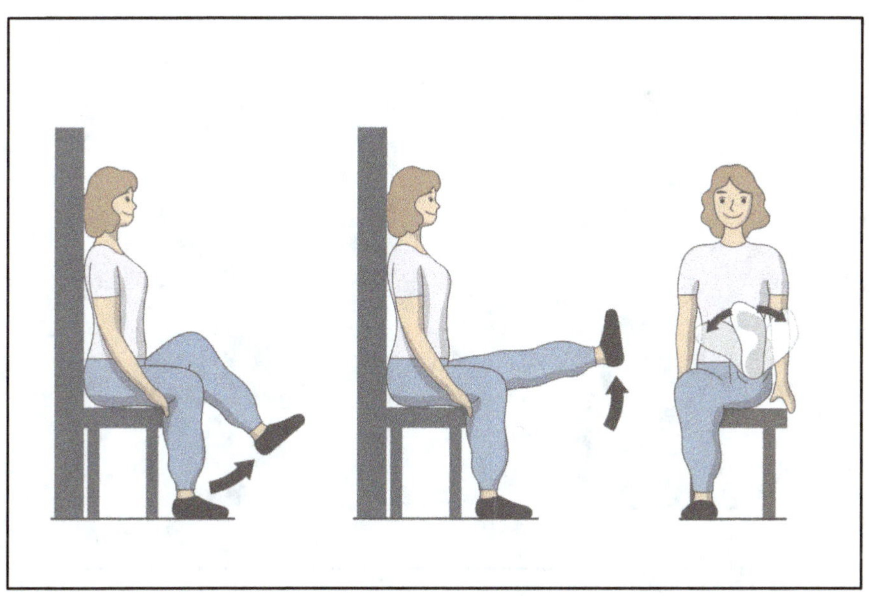

4. Heel Alignment

a. Sit up straight in a chair with your hands resting lightly on your hips.
b. Bring your legs and feet together.
c. Slowly spread your legs apart, keeping your heels together, until your feet are aligned with your heels touching each other.
d. Hold this position for 10 seconds, then slowly bring your legs and feet back together.
e. Feel the muscles inside your thighs working and repeat this 10 times.

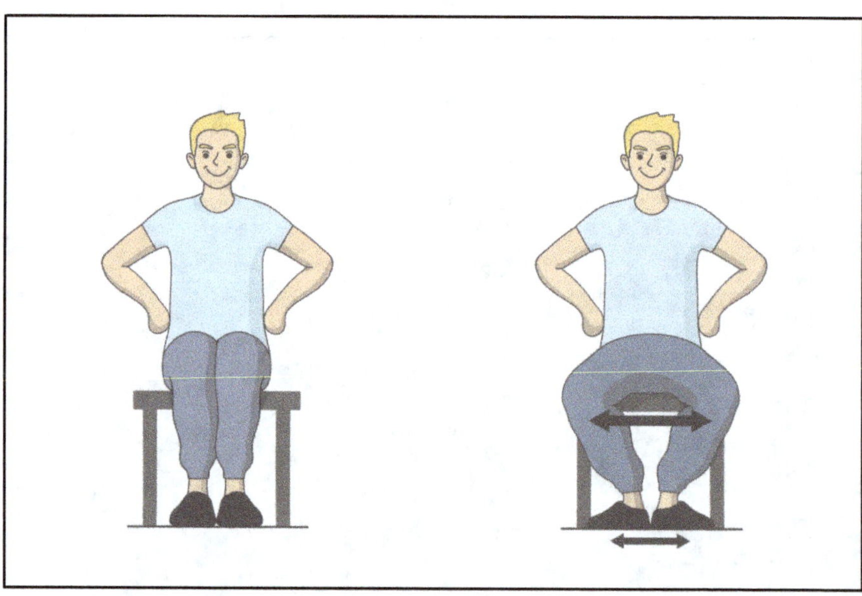

5. Seated Wall Push

a. Sit facing a wall and place your hands on the wall as if you are pushing it.
b. Keep your gaze level and your back straight.
c. Push against the wall, ensuring your chair doesn't slide back.
d. Bend your elbows and hold for 10 seconds.
e. Repeat this movement 10 times.

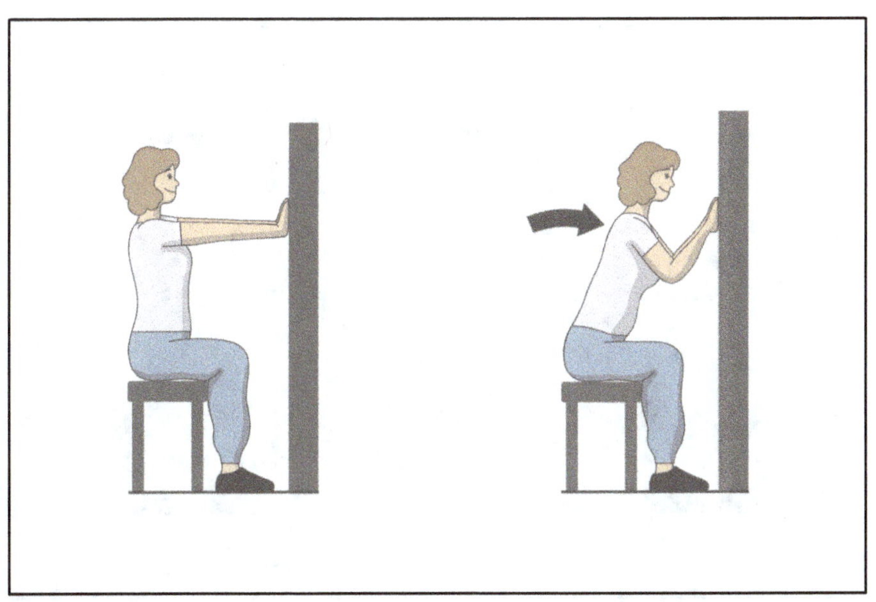

6. Side Stretch with Interlaced Fingers

a. Sit up straight, interlace your fingers, and place your hands behind your head.
b. Look straight ahead and hold for 10 seconds.
c. Bend your body to the right, feeling the stretch, and hold for 10 seconds.
d. Return to the center, then bend to the left and hold for 10 seconds.
e. Repeat these side stretches 10 times, feeling the movement in your waist.

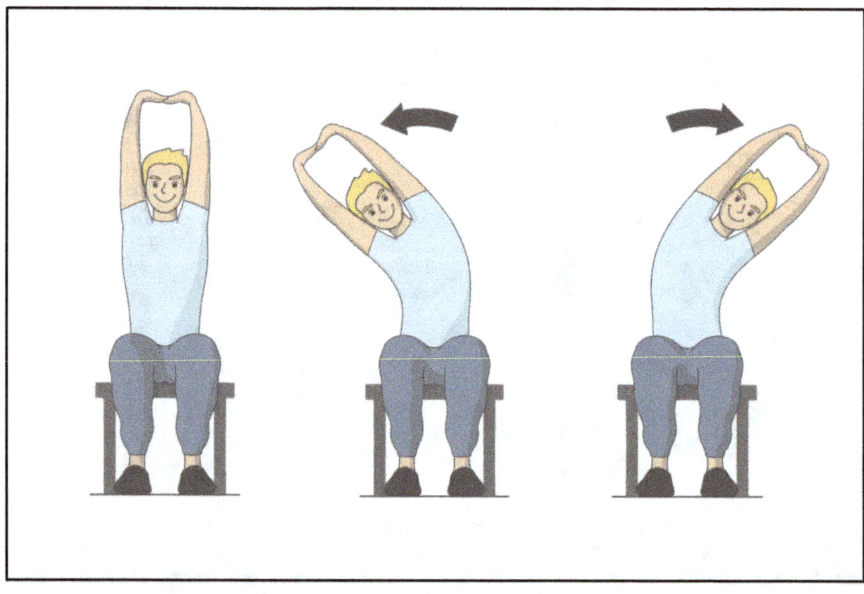

Six Lying Down Exercises

1. Upper Abdominal Crunch

a. Lie on your back with your hands raised above your head and your legs lifted to a right angle.
b. Raise your upper body, reaching your hands towards your feet.
c. Hold this position for 10 seconds, then return to the starting position.
d. Feel the tension in your upper abdominal muscles and repeat 10 times.

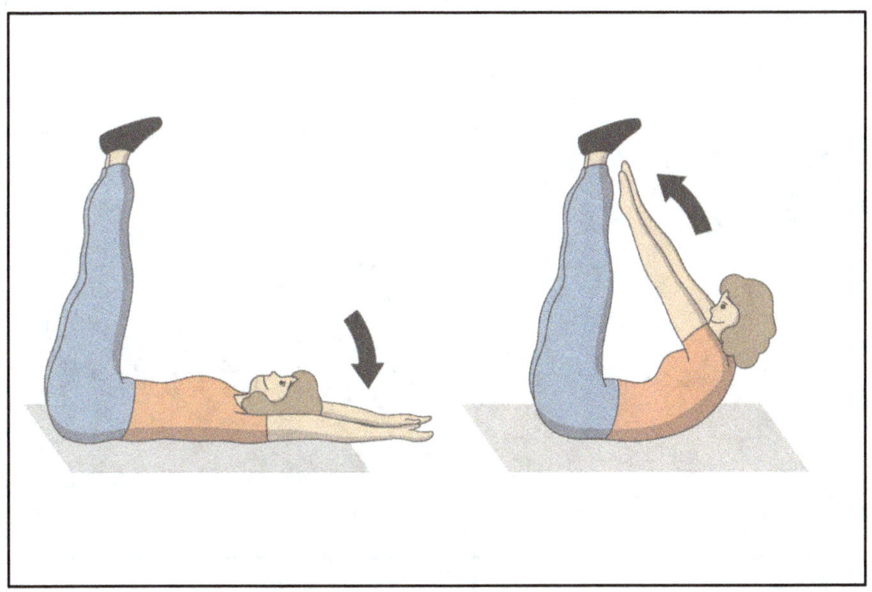

2. Cobra Stretch

a. Lie face down with your elbows bent and hands placed near your shoulders.
b. Push the ground with your palms and slowly lift your upper body.
c. Hold this position for 10 seconds, then slowly lower yourself back down.
d. Be careful not to strain your back; perform within a comfortable range.
e. This stretch helps correct a hunched back and inwardly curved pelvis.

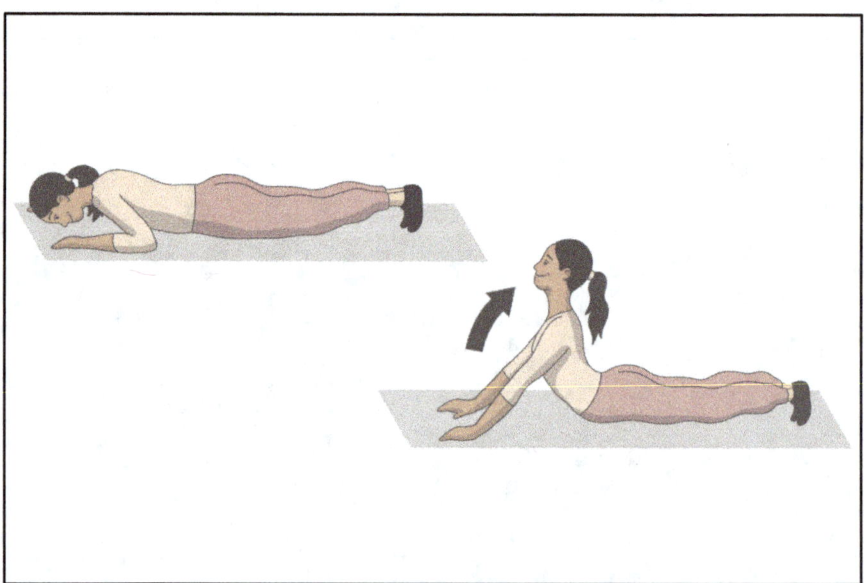

3. Scissor Leg Lifts

a. Lie on your side in a straight line, supporting yourself with one arm.
b. Focus on your thighs and sides, lifting your leg at a 30-40 degree angle.
c. Hold for 10 seconds, then return to the starting position.
d. Repeat this 10 times, then switch legs.

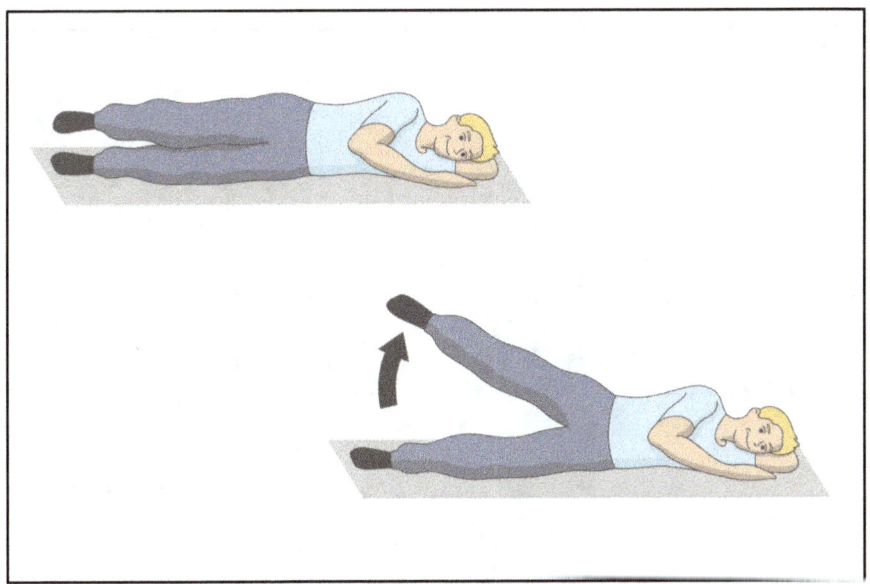

4. Chest Opener

a. Fold a thick blanket and place it from your head to your hips, then lie on it.
b. Position your legs hip-width apart and bend your knees at a right angle to the floor.
c. Raise your arms to a right angle and hold for 10 seconds.
d. Slowly lower your hands and elbows to the floor outside your chest.
e. Repeat this 10 times, feeling the stretch in your shoulders and chest.

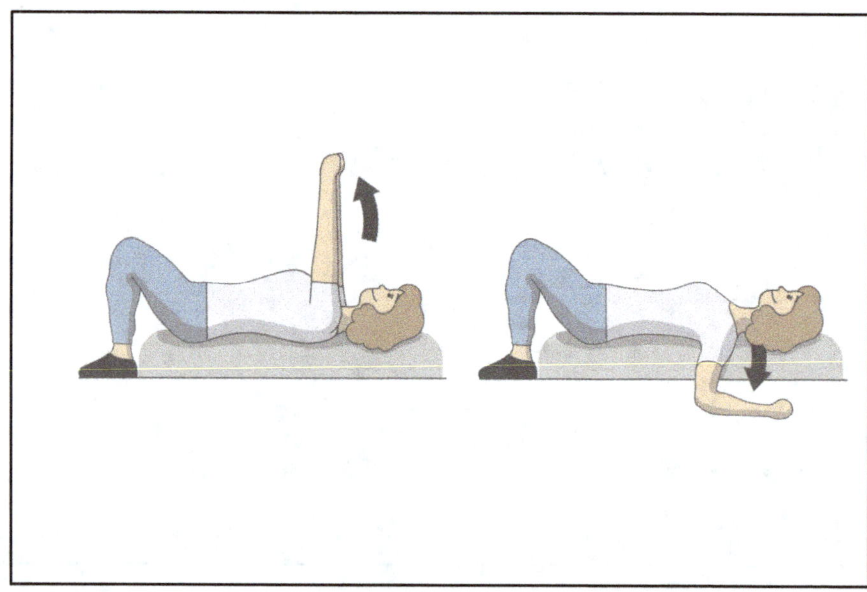

5. Prone Thigh Lift

a. Lie face down with a pillow or towel under your belly.
b. Stretch your legs out and bend your right leg at a right angle.
c. Slowly lift your bent right thigh and hold for 10 seconds.
d. Lower your leg slowly, feeling the strength in your glutes, and repeat 5 times before switching legs.
e. This exercise strengthens your glutes, back, and core muscles.

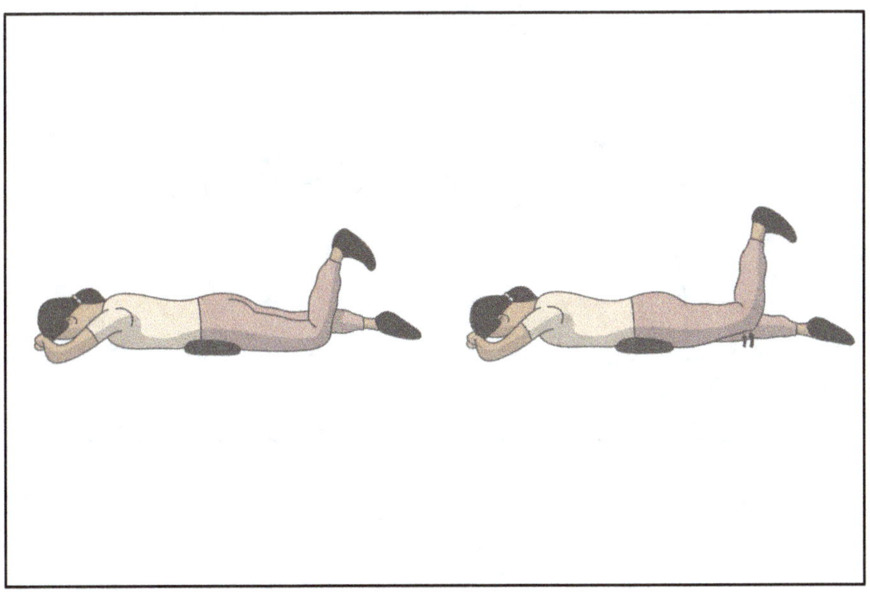

6. Stretching Like a Starfish

a. Lie flat on your back with your arms and legs extended.
b. Stretch your arms above your head in a straight line.
c. Press your back against the floor and hold for 10 seconds.
d. Repeat this stretch 10 times.

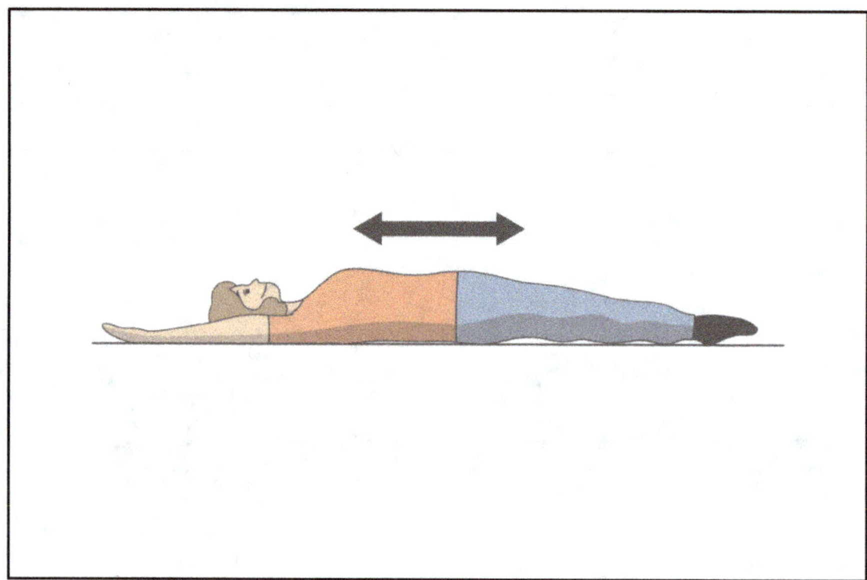

7. HEALTHY HABITS WITH EXERCISE: SLEEP WELL, EAT WELL, LAUGH WELL

Sleep Well: Use blackout curtains, avoid smartphones before bed.
Eat Well: Eat a balanced diet, enjoy your meals, chew slowly.
Laugh Well: You don't laugh because you're happy; you're happy because you laugh.

As we start incorporating exercise into our routine, we also need to adjust other lifestyle habits. There are three key habits to focus on: sleeping well, eating well, and laughing well.

Many people struggle with sleep. Insomnia is a common issue not only for Parkinson's patients but for many people in the modern age. To sleep well, we need to create an environment conducive to good sleep. The most important factor is blocking out light. Before the advent of electricity, our ancestors' daily patterns were dependent on sunlight. They slept when it got dark and woke up when it was light, maintaining a harmonious sleep-wake cycle. Nowadays, there is too much light. While bright environments have their benefits, they are not good for insomnia. To signal to our brain that it's time to sleep, we need to block out light. If you live in a brightly lit area, use blackout curtains to prevent street lights from shining in through the window.

Also, avoid bright lights at least an hour before bed. Smartphones and televisions emit very bright light. You might have experienced seeing images from a video you watched before bed reappear in your dreams. Before falling asleep, our eyes need to be free from intense light stimulation. Watching TV or videos on a smartphone before bed is not good for sleep. Turn off the lights, phones, and TV, and minimize light exposure to fall asleep. However, for safety, keeping a few dim, soft lights on is fine.

Secondly, we need to eat well. A well-prepared meal is better than any medicine.

"What should I eat?"

Many Parkinson's patients ask this question. A diet rich in vegetables and greens is very beneficial for Parkinson's disease as it helps prevent constipation. Avoid greasy, sweet, and salty foods. However, it is important to consume adequate protein, alternating between meat and fish. Parkinson's patients tend to lose weight easily, so they need to consume enough calories. Don't just make quick meals like grabbing a microwave dinner. Even if you don't have a variety of side dishes, aim for a balanced diet each day, savoring your food and chewing slowly. Eating well is also crucial for exercising.

Thirdly, let's laugh well. I once attended a laughter therapy lecture. The therapist kept telling the audience to laugh even if it felt forced. Even though it wasn't funny, eventually, it became genuinely amusing. It also improved my mood. Our brain is simple; it assumes we are happy if we laugh. The way to live joyfully is to believe that you are happy. Surround yourself with positive news and happy people. Today, we are bombarded with information. In the past, we had morning newspapers and the 9 o'clock news, but now endless information flows from our smartphones. Avoid news that makes you angry. Listening to fun and touching stories is enough for a fulfilling life. Don't stress over things that haven't happened yet. Break free from the whirlwind of online videos and resist the bombardment of unsolicited clips. Online content tends to become more biased the more you engage with it. Parkinson's patients need to stimulate their brains in diverse ways. Focusing too much on one thing is not good for brain health.

8. HOW TO EXERCISE WHEN MEDICATION WEARS OFF

When Parkinson's patients first start taking medication, the effects last a long time. However, as the disease progresses, the effect of levodopa diminishes more quickly. The period when the medication is effective is called 'on' time, and when it wears off, it's called 'off' time. Just like a light switch turning on and off, the medication's effect can come and go.

If you experience on-off fluctuations, consult your neurologist first. Adjusting your Parkinson's medication is the primary approach to managing these fluctuations. Sometimes, the medication is switched to a long-acting formulation, or the dosage is increased. Keeping a Parkinson's diary to track medication times, effectiveness, and when it wears off can greatly help in adjusting your medication. If you experience on-off fluctuations, make sure to keep a Parkinson's diary.

"How should I exercise during on-off fluctuations?"

Exercise during 'on' times when the medication is effective. Active exercise should always be done during these periods. During 'off' times when the medication wears off, patiently wait until the medication kicks in again. Exercising during 'off' times can be physically and mentally demanding, increasing the risk of joint injuries and falls. Therefore, start exercising when the medication is fully effective.

To schedule your exercise, you need to know when the medication is effective for you. Know how long it takes for the medication to kick in after you take it, how long it lasts, and when it starts to wear off. Keeping a Parkinson's diary is essential for this. When undergoing rehabilitation therapy, ensure it's done during 'on' times. If you go out, carry extra Parkinson's medication to prepare for sudden drops in effectiveness.

9. MY BODY MOVES ON ITS OWN: EXERCISING WITH DYSKINESIA

Dyskinesia, a common late-stage side effect of Parkinson's medication, often accompanies the on-off phenomenon previously described. Dyskinesia makes your body move involuntarily. It might feel like you're twisting your torso back and forth, or your arms and legs might move in a wavy, uncontrolled manner. These movements typically occur when the medication is at its strongest. When the medication's effect wears off, the dyskinesia subsides, and you return to a more still state.

Earlier, I advised exercising during 'on' times when the medication is effective. However, dyskinesia might also be present during these times.

"How should I exercise if I have severe dyskinesia?"
"Is it even safe to exercise?"

Research indicates that intensive rehabilitation exercise therapy is effective for Parkinson's patients with dyskinesia. In studies, patients who underwent rehabilitation exercises showed improvement in all aspects of Parkinson's symptoms, including dyskinesia.
Patients were divided into two groups. One group received intensive therapy focusing on walking, balance, and strength, while the other group received general physical therapy. Both groups showed improvement, but the intensive therapy group showed slightly better results. Exercise remains a beneficial choice even with dyskinesia. In fact, movement irregularities often lessen during exercise.

If you exercise with dyskinesia, keep three things in mind:

First, be extra careful to maintain balance. Dyskinesia can cause you to lose balance as your torso and neck move or your legs move erratically, increasing the risk of falls.

Second, don't forcefully try to stop the involuntary movements or move excessively to hide them. Let the movements happen naturally. If you need to perform a specific action, consciously and repeatedly guide your brain to maintain that action. Even with the same movement, intending to perform it accurately helps signal your brain.

Third, be cautious to avoid injuries. Involuntary movements can cause your arms or legs to hit objects, leading to injuries. Keep your surroundings clean and clear, especially paths where you might trip. Avoid paths with large stones or uneven surfaces where you could easily fall.

Patients with dyskinesia often feel more self-conscious and may become more withdrawn. It's understandable, as the constant movement can draw attention. If you're hesitant to go out for exercise, try dancing to music at home. Dancing is highly recommended for all Parkinson's patients and is especially suitable for those with dyskinesia. Dancing can help you embrace the freedom of movement. Follow a dance routine or just dance freely—both are great exercises and help relieve the burden of structured movements.

There's no need to limit exercise because of dyskinesia. In fact, stay active and keep exercising. Remember to eat well, as dyskinesia increases energy expenditure, potentially leading to significant weight loss. Drink plenty of water slowly and maintain a balanced diet.

10. EXERCISE FOR WALKING DIFFICULTIES

Among the various symptoms of Parkinson's disease, let's take another look at walking difficulties. When you have walking difficulties, many exercises become limited. So, how should you deal with it? First, you need to be aware. Remember that you have postural instability and walking difficulties. Postural instability, a bit of a complex term, can be simply referred to as "balance issues." When your balance is impaired and you have walking difficulties, you need to be particularly cautious. While you might feel like you want to run everywhere like you did in your twenties, being hasty is the worst thing for walking difficulties because it can lead to accidents.

Accidents can happen from falling or from slipping off a bed or chair. Or you might slip in the bathroom and get hurt. If it's just a bruise or a minor cut, consider yourself lucky. But many of our patients also have osteoporosis, and their muscles and ligaments are weak. Falling can result in broken arms or legs. Sometimes, hitting your head during a fall can cause traumatic brain injury. In fact, one of the biggest reasons for hospitalization in nursing homes or care facilities is falls. Many patients with Parkinson's disease who were doing well end up in facilities once they start having mobility issues. Surgery due to injuries also exposes you to many risks. So, if you've started falling, it's crucial to be extra cautious—this cannot be emphasized enough.

Creating a Safe Environment

Make the patient's surroundings safe. Chairs with wheels are dangerous. When sitting down, the lack of strength and balance control can make you plop down suddenly. A wheeled chair can move, causing you to fall. All chairs should be sturdy and stable, so they don't move when sitting down or getting up. Pathways you frequently use should be non-slip and free of tripping hazards. If there's a step, mark it with colored tape to make it more visible. If falls are severe, install safety bars on walls to hold onto while moving. Choose flooring materials that can cushion a fall. Especially in the bathroom, where falls are common, install grab bars near the toilet for support when sitting down and standing up. Just like child-proofing a home with safety sponges on furniture edges, inspect your home for places where you could fall and get hurt, and take precautions.

"Is there no medication for this?"

Unfortunately, there is no medication that significantly improves postural instability and walking difficulties. If the dosage of levodopa is too low, balance and walking can worsen. In advanced Parkinson's disease, the medication's effect can suddenly wear off, a phenomenon known as "off" periods, which can lead to freezing episodes. Overall, when medication levels are low, balance and walking can be particularly difficult. If balance and walking become more challenging, it may be necessary to increase the dosage of dopamine-related Parkinson's medications to an appropriate level. If symptoms do not improve despite increasing dopamine medication sufficiently, further increasing the dosage may not be very helpful.

"Will surgery help?"

As mentioned in the section on surgical treatments, these symptoms do not respond well to Deep Brain Stimulation (DBS) surgery. So, if postural instability and walking difficulties are more severe than other symptoms, DBS surgery may not be suitable. Recently, there have been experimental attempts with different surgical areas, showing some improvement in postural instability. Hopefully, we will see good results soon.

"What kind of exercise should I do?"

Freezing is when you suddenly stop walking and feel like you are stuck in place. Patients with freezing can use various cues and tricks to overcome it. Try walking while loudly counting "One, two, one, two" or saying "Right foot, left foot." You can also walk to the rhythm of music or a metronome. Practice stepping over the patterns on the pavement, one step at a time. If you use a cane, point it forward to guide your steps. These tricks can help you keep walking continuously.

Emphasizing the need to be cautious about falling can often lead to the question: Should I just stay in bed and not exercise? Absolutely not. You should continue to exercise in some way. Just do it safely. It's best to use assistive devices or have someone help you. You might wear protective gear and undergo robot-assisted therapy. This helps keep your muscles and joints in a condition where they can still move.

11. ANOTHER COMPANION: THE ROLE OF THE CAREGIVER

The Caregiver's Story

"My husband was diagnosed with Parkinson's disease two years ago."

"Even before the diagnosis, he had several troubling symptoms, but the two years following the diagnosis have been extremely challenging. Of course, the shock was greatest for my husband, the patient. But as a caregiver, I don't know how to help him."

"I worry that I might be doing something wrong, making his condition worse."

Just hearing the name Parkinson's disease is a huge shock. The disease starts slowly. At some point when symptoms become noticeable, you might hear a doctor say, "It's Parkinson's disease." The psychological burden of the name "Parkinson's" is immense. Your body may not feel much different than it did the day before the diagnosis, but your mind feels like it has plunged into a deep pit. This isn't just the story of a few sensitive and fragile people; it's what most patients go through. Life before and after the Parkinson's diagnosis feels distinctly different, not because your body suddenly worsened, but because the name Parkinson's started weighing heavily on your mind.

This emotional burden is no less for caregivers. Caregivers also experience shock, especially if it's someone you rely on and believe in who is now ill. It can feel even more devastating than for the patient. As a caregiver for someone with Parkinson's disease, you feel a significant responsibility. The role of the caregiver in Parkinson's disease is crucial.

First, the caregiver is a "companion."

"Companion" is a more fitting term than "caregiver." A companion is someone who has been there before the diagnosis and stays by the patient's side during the diagnosis and treatment process. They share the patient's emotions first and feel the tough symptoms alongside them. A companion walks the Parkinson's journey together. The path won't always be smooth. Sometimes you'll walk comfortably on a wide road, other times you might stumble on a rocky path. You may feel like you're at a dead end, about to fall off a cliff, but then a new path opens up ahead.

As a caregiver, your responsibility is significant. But you don't have to carry the patient all the way from start to finish. You're there to help them up when they fall and discuss the best way forward. The role of the caregiver isn't to shoulder all the daily responsibilities alone. The most important thing for a companion is to be there and walk the path together. That alone makes you an excellent companion.

Second, you need to understand Parkinson's disease well.

There will be many moments during the patient's symptoms and treatment process where decisions need to be made. Situations will arise where the patient cannot decide alone. At those times, it helps to have a good understanding of Parkinson's disease. Observe and understand the patient's symptoms and changes in daily life. The caregiver's perspective can greatly assist communication with the doctor during medical consultations.

These days, the conditions for studying are excellent. There's a wealth of information available. However, too much information can be overwhelming and confusing. Avoid becoming fixated on biased information. While it's important to study Parkinson's disease, stick to well-established medical resources and proven books or websites. This will help you steer your course as a caregiver more effectively.

Third, caregivers also need support.

In many cases, caregivers are the closest family members. In turn, the patient's emotions are often projected onto those family members. When the patient feels physically unwell or depressed, they may become irritable and lash out at their caregivers. People tend to blame someone else when they feel weak, and the easiest target is often the family member closest to them. You might think, "The patient must be having a hard time; I need to be patient and understanding." But while your mind understands, your heart might feel like it's breaking. After holding it in for so long, you might finally snap and yell at the patient, then feel guilty for not being more understanding.

As a doctor, my primary concern is the patient, but I also deeply value the caregiver. Caregivers are also human and need support. If you focus solely on the patient 24/7, you will easily become exhausted. I often see caregivers struggling with stress, depression, sleep disorders, and anxiety. While you play the role of "the patient's caregiver," your own life and well-being are also precious and important. Spend time in your own space, take time for yourself, and maintain your own life. If you feel mentally strained, seek treatment. Build a network of people who can support you. Let go of some of the burden of responsibility, guilt, and the sadness of difficult situations. You cannot solve everything or carry all the weight alone. Just walking alongside the patient as a companion is already fulfilling a significant role.

"Take care of your own body and mind. That's also a way to help the patient."

CONCLUSION

Parkinson's disease progresses slowly. It can be incredibly distressing when you feel like your symptoms aren't improving. You might think, "I could walk well last year, but now my legs feel heavy and I can hardly move," causing you to worry deeply. The thought that you might end up like the advanced Parkinson's patients you see on TV can be very disheartening and drain your motivation.

But take a moment to look up and see the world around you. Every living being follows the same path. The flowers that bloom so brilliantly, the mighty oak tree standing tall, and the tiger roaring majestically all eventually fade according to the laws of nature. Parkinson's disease is just a condition that speeds up the aging process a bit. It's simply experiencing what everyone goes through, just a little sooner.

We cannot predict the future, but we have today. So, let's smile our biggest smile in the present moment. Lift yourself from feelings of helplessness and depression. Focus not on what you can't do, but on what you can still enjoy doing. Enjoy every small step and the biggest laughter you can muster. Mr. Parkinson, let's walk together.

REFERENCES

Part 1

LEWIS, C.H.E.R.R.Y.(2018). Enlightened mr. Parkinson: The Pioneering Life of a forgotten English surgeon. Amazon. Retrieved April 17, 2023, https://www.amazon.com/Enlightened-Mr-Parkinson-Pioneering-Forgotten/dp/1681774542

Ji-Young Kim, Han-Joon Kim, Beom S.Jeon. Prevalence and characteristics of nonmotor symptoms in Krean Parkinson's disease patients and its relationship with experience of alternative therapies. Korean journal of neurological association, 2013, 31(1): 8-14.

Kumar, N. (2009). The Sydney Multicenter Study of Parkinson's Disease: The inevitability of dementia at 20 years. Yearbook of Neurology and Neurosurgery, 2009, 94–95.

Part 2

Caspersen, C.J., Powell, K.E., &Christenson, G.M. (1985). Physical activity, exercise, and physical fitness:definitions and distinctions for health-related research. Public Health Report, 1985, 100(2): 126-131.

Cilia, R., Akpalu, A., Sarfo, F. S., Cham, M., Amboni, M., Cereda, E., Fabbri, M., Adjei, P., Akassi, J., Bonetti, A., & Pezzoli, G. (2014). The modern pre-levodopa era of parkinson's disease: Insights into motor complications from sub-Saharan africa. Brain, 137(10), 2731–2742.

Gosvig, C. F., Kjaer, S. K., Blaakær, J., Høgdall, E., Høgdall, C., & Jensen, A. (2015). Coffee, tea, and caffeine consumption and risk of epithelial ovarian cancer and borderline ovarian tumors: Results from a Danish case-control study. Acta Oncologica, 54(8), 1144–1151.

Hernán, M. A., Takkouche, B., Caamaño-Isorna, F., & Gestal-Otero, J. J. (2002). A meta-analysis of coffee drinking, cigarette smoking, and the risk of parkinson's disease. Annals of Neurology, 52(3), 276–284.

Kumar, N. (2009). The Sydney Multicenter Study of Parkinson's Disease: The inevitability of dementia at 20 years. Yearbook of Neurology and Neurosurgery, 2009, 94–95.

LEWIS, C. H. E. R. R. Y. (2018). Enlightened mr. Parkinson: The Pioneering Life of a forgotten English surgeon. Amazon. Retrieved April 17, 2023, from https://www.amazon.com/Enlightened-Mr-Parkinson-Pioneering-Forgotten/dp/1681774542

Paul, K. C., Chuang, Y. H., Shih, I. F., Keener, A., Bordelon, Y., Bronstein, J. M., & Ritz, B. (2019). The association between lifestyle factors and parkinson's disease progression and mortality. Movement Disorders, 34(1), 58–66.

Wirdefeldt, K., Gatz, M., Pawitan, Y., & Pedersen, N. L. (2004). Risk and protective factors for parkinson's disease: A study in Swedish twins. Annals of Neurology, 57(1), 27–33.

Zhang, W., Deng, B., Xie, F., Zhou, H., Guo, J.-F., Jiang, H., Sim, A., Tang, B., & Wang, Q. (2022). Efficacy of repetitive transcranial magnetic stimulation in parkinson's disease: A systematic review and meta-analysis of Randomised Controlled Trials. EClinicalMedicine, 52, 101589.

Part 3

Amara, A. W., Chahine, L., Seedorff, N., Caspell-Garcia, C. J., Coffey, C., & Simuni, T. (2019). Self-reported physical activity levels and clinical progression in early parkinson's disease. Parkinsonism & Related Disorders, 61, 118–125.

Amara, A. W., Wood, K. H., Joop, A., Memon, R. A., Pilkington, J., Tuggle, S. C., Reams, J., Barrett, M. J., Edwards, D. A., Weltman, A. L., Hurt, C. P., Cutter, G., & Bamman, M. M. (2020). Randomized, controlled trial of exercise on objective and subjective sleep in parkinson's disease. Movement Disorders, 35(6), 947–958.

Cohen, A. D., Tillerson, J. L., Smith, A. D., Schallert, T., & Zigmond, M. J. (2003). Neuroprotective effects of prior limb use in 6-hydroxy-dopamine-treated rats: Possible role of GDNF. Journal of Neurochemistry, 85(2), 299–305.

Corrigendum: Exercise builds brain health: Key roles of growth factor cascades and inflammation. (2007). Trends in Neurosciences, 30(10), 489.

da Silva, F. C., Iop, R. da, de Oliveira, L. C., Boll, A. M., de Alvarenga, J. G., Gutierres Filho, P. J., de Melo, L. M., Xavier, A. J., & da Silva, R. (2018). Effects of physical exercise programs on cognitive function in parkinson's disease patients: A systematic review of randomized controlled trials of the last 10 years. PLOS ONE, 13(2).

Fox, C., Ramig, L., Ciucci, M., Sapir, S., McFarland, D., & Farley, B. (2006). The science and practice of LSVT/Loud: Neural plasticity-principled approach to treating individuals with parkinson disease and other neurological disorders. Seminars in Speech and Language, 27(4), 283–299.

Hallal, P. C., Andersen, L. B., Bull, F. C., Guthold, R., Haskell, W., & Ekelund, U. (2012). Global physical activity levels: Surveillance progress, pitfalls, and prospects. The Lancet, 380(9838), 247–257.

Lauzé, M., Daneault, J.-F., & Duval, C. (2016). The effects of physical activity in parkinson's disease: A Review. Journal of Parkinson's Disease, 6(4), 685–698.

Lord, S., Godfrey, A., Galna, B., Mhiripiri, D., Burn, D., & Rochester, L. (2013). Ambulatory activity in Incident parkinson's: More than meets the eye? Journal of Neurology, 260(12), 2964–2972.

Martinez-Martin, P., Rodriguez-Blazquez, C., Kurtis, M. M., & Chaudhuri, K. R. (2011). The impact of non-motor symptoms on health-related quality of life of patients with parkinson's disease. Movement Disorders, 26(3), 399–406.

Monteiro-Junior, R. S., Cevada, T., Oliveira, B. R. R., Lattari, E., Portugal, E. M. M., Carvalho, A., & Deslandes, A. C. (2015). We need to move more: Neurobiological hypotheses of physical exercise as a treatment for parkinson's disease. Medical Hypotheses, 85(5), 537–541.

Oguh, O., Eisenstein, A., Kwasny, M., & Simuni, T. (2014). Back to the basics: Regular exercise matters in parkinson's disease: Results from the National Parkinson Foundation QII Registry Study. Parkinsonism & Related Disorders, 20(11), 1221–1225.

The study that could change everything. Home | Parkinson's Progression Markers Initiative. (n.d.). Retrieved April 17, 2023, from https://www.ppmi-info.org/

Sutoo, D., & Akiyama, K. (2003). Regulation of brain function by exercise. Neurobiology of Disease, 13(1), 1–14.

Tillerson, J. L., Caudle, W. M., Reverón, M. E., & Miller, G. W. (2003). Exercise induces behavioral recovery and attenuates neurochemical deficits in rodent models of parkinson's disease. Neuroscience, 119(3), 899–911.

Tillerson, J. L., Cohen, A. D., Philhower, J., Miller, G. W., Zigmond, M. J., & Schallert, T. (2001). Forced limb-use effects on the behavioral and neurochemical effects of 6-hydroxydopamine. The Journal of Neuroscience, 21(12), 4427–4435.

Tomlinson, C. L., Patel, S., Meek, C., Herd, C. P., Clarke, C. E., Stowe, R., Shah, L., Sackley, C. M., Deane, K. H. O., Wheatley, K., & Ives, N. (2013). Physiotherapy versus placebo or no intervention in parkinson's disease. Cochrane Database of Systematic Reviews.

Xu, Q., Park, Y., Huang, X., Hollenbeck, A., Blair, A., Schatzkin, A., & Chen, H. (2010). Physical activities and future risk of parkinson disease. Neurology, 75(4), 341–348.

Yang, F., Trolle Lagerros, Y., Bellocco, R., Adami, H.-O., Fang, F., Pedersen, N. L., & Wirdefeldt, K. (2014). Physical activity and risk of parkinson's disease in the Swedish National March cohort. Brain, 138(2), 269–275.